LIVE 10 HEALTHY YEARS LONGER

LIVE 10 HEALTHY YEARS LONGER

JAN W. KUZMA AND CECIL MURPHEY

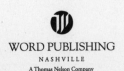

WORD PUBLISHING

NASHVILLE

A Thomas Nelson Company

Unless otherwise indicated, Scripture quotations used in this book are from the Holy Bible, New International Version® (NIV). Copyright © 1973, 1978, 1984, International Bible Society. Used by permission of Zondervan Bible Publishers. Other Scripture references are from the following sources:

The New King James Version (NKJV), copyright © 1979, 1980, 1982, Thomas Nelson, Inc., Publishers.

The Revised Standard Version of the Bible (RSV). Copyright © 1946, 1952, 1971, 1973 by the Division of Christian Education of the National Council of the Churches of Christ in the USA. Used by permission.

The New Revised Standard Version Bible (NRSV), © 1989 by the Division of Christian Education of the National Council of the Churches of Christ in the USA.

The Contemporary English Version (CEV) © 1991 by the American Bible Society. Used by permission.

The Holy Bible, New Living Translation (NLT), copyright © 1996. Used by permission of Tyndale House Publishers, Inc., Wheaton, Illinois 60189. All rights reserved.

The information in this book provides a general overview of health-related topics and may not apply to everyone. To find out if this information applies to you and to get more information about any health-related issue, talk to your family doctor. The health claims stated in this book are those of the authors. Neither Word Publishing nor Thomas Nelson expresses any opinion as to the validity of those health claims.

Library of Congress Cataloging-in-Publication Data

Kuzma, Jan W.

    Live ten healthy years longer/by Jan W. Kuzma and Cecil Murphey.

       p. cm.

    ISBN 0-8499-3770-1

    1. Longevity. 2. Health. 3. Aging. I. Title: Live 10 healthy years longer. II. Murphey, Cecil B. III. Title.

    RA776.75 .K89 2000

    613—dc21

99-045953

CIP

CONTENTS

ACKNOWLEDGMENTS

Jan Kuzma thanks Dr. Frank R. Lemon, who introduced him to the field of biostatistics and to Loma Linda University, and Dr. Mervin G. Hardinge, his respected dean, who offered him his first position in the School of Public Health. He also thanks Dr. Roland L. Phillips, a college classmate and fellow researcher at Loma Linda University. Together they submitted the first grant application to fund the Adventist Health Study, and when it was funded, Dr. Phillips became its first director.

Jan and Cec also thank their wives, Kay Kuzma, who offers Jan daily inspiration, and Shirley Murphey, Cec's devoted editor and wonderful partner.

"HOW LONG WOULD YOU LIKE TO LIVE?"

CHAPTER 1

RICHARD CLARK'S doctor first asked him how long he'd like to live when Richard was thirty-five years old, a time when he had just begun to notice his decreased energy level. Hefty love handles had appeared around his middle and loaded him down with an extra 25 pounds. Tiny crow's-feet had started to appear around his eyes. "Hmm, how long would I like to live?" Richard repeated. "Until I'm about eighty-five or ninety—if I can still be in good health."

. . .

"But if you're not in good health," came the second question, "then how long would you want to live?"

"Then I'm not sure," he said. "Not that long anyway."

Richard Clark also became aware that his blood pressure was slightly elevated, and his doctor warned him not to allow his cholesterol level to get any higher. Despite his doctor's advice, Richard didn't quit smoking. He did admit that he knew he should give up cigarettes. But, like many American males who feel no pain or discomfort, he paid little attention to the warning signs of his declining health. As he had done all his adult life, Richard Clark continued to make decisions about his lifestyle—most of them unconsciously.

This week Richard Clark turned fifty-five. Although he doesn't know it yet, he is preparing for an early death. If he's extremely lucky, he'll live to age sixty-five. But the odds are stacked against him. He did quit smoking five years ago, which has helped. For fifty-five years, however, Richard has been preparing to die of a catastrophic illness: heart disease, cancer, or stroke.

Carol Clark, Richard's wife, doesn't know it yet, but she will survive him by six years—*maybe*. If she's really lucky, she will live until she's seventy-one. At age fifty-two, Carol is acutely aware of the 40 extra pounds she carries on her 5'4" frame. She has successfully dieted nine times in the past five years. After each diet, however, she ballooned back to her original weight and gained four or five additional pounds before she started the next regimen. Even though she isn't aware of the adverse health effects of her many diets and her lifestyle, Carol is also preparing to die of a catastrophic illness.

Although women can look forward to living six more years than men, the average American male can expect to reach the age of seventy-two. Not everyone, of course, will live to the "average" age. Many die much younger!

Sounds a little bleak, doesn't it?

But this doesn't have to be a picture of you.

You don't have to be an average statistic.

You can beat those statistics and live healthier, longer, and happier for another decade.

You can make that happen.

But will you?

Would you make sensible changes in your lifestyle if it enabled you to live nine or ten years longer—and healthier at the same time? Would you like to enjoy the golden years without physical restrictions? to have more vitality? to perform better as you advance in age?

In contrast to the Clarks, consider Joe and Vicki Nichols. On his fortieth birthday, Joe had a complete physical. The results forced him to take stock of himself. He joined a health spa primarily to lose 50 pounds. He also learned to play tennis and became fairly good at the game. To improve his breathing, Joe dumped his pack-a-day habit of smoking. He never went on a weight-loss diet—he didn't have to. He dropped nearly 60 pounds over a two-year period. By his forty-second birthday, Joe had drastically altered his lifestyle. His once-racing pulse hit a steady 70 beats a minute; his cholesterol level consistently hovered at 185.

Vicki, who was in worse shape than Joe, reluctantly cooperated with her husband's lifestyle changes. Despite her misgivings, she learned to cook differently and found it an exciting adventure. "I kept learning new things," she said. Even with a hereditary factor for high blood pressure, lifestyle changes enabled Vicki to stop taking medication and maintain a pressure of 135/80.

The best news about Joe and Vicki is that he is now eighty-four and she is eighty-six. "My bones feel a little creaky in the mornings," Joe says, "but after Vicki and I do our two-mile walk and a few exercises, I feel all right." Neither is on any medication. Vicki's weight, she says, "is about six pounds more than I would prefer it to be, but I don't plan to do anything about it."

Obviously, Joe and Vicki have already beaten the statistics.

They aren't that unusual.

Thousands of others who have altered their lifestyles have begun to enjoy better health and longer life.

You could be a Vicki or a Joe!

We hope that sounds exciting. It is possible, and it's not as difficult as you may think, although it does require some work. You will have to make a few simple changes in your life.

As you think about what you have read so far, ask yourself the following questions. Would you like to

- live into your eighties—even into your nineties?
- be/stay in good physical health during those years?
- remain mentally alert all your life?
- be of normal weight without dieting?

- feel good about yourself?

- enjoy each day of your life?

- release negative stress and live a calmer life?

If you answered yes to these questions, did you also wonder whether these things were achievable? Did you have trouble thinking of yourself as attaining all of them? Do they seem like impossible goals?

Or did you assume that even though others live well and long, this book probably doesn't apply to you? Did you remember too many diet and physical fitness failures you've suffered?

That was the past.

Your future doesn't have to be a repeat of failure.

You can turn every one of these questions into positive statements about your life. Thousands have already put into practice the principles that promote a healthier lifestyle, which has enabled them to live longer and more productively.

Before you start to scoff, we want to tell you that these people are not only healthier and alive longer, but the evidence indicates that they also

- feel good about who they are

- enjoy life

- have a positive outlook

- accept responsibility for their health

- honor their bodies as God's holy temple and keep them in good condition

Throughout this book you'll learn information and receive encouragement to help you opt for longer and healthier living. Because of extensive research, we can prove that right now—today—at least a million Americans have learned the secrets of healthy longevity.

These secrets can be yours as well.

They're not unfounded boasts, unrealistic claims, or speculation. They aren't theories or vague projections. We can verify the secrets revealed in this book.

In 1960, under the direction of Dr. Frank Lemon, Loma Linda University began an ongoing study in cooperation with the American Cancer Society. Dr. Lemon and his team enlisted 27,514 people. The initial objective was to compare them with one million randomly selected Californians to determine the factors associated with the development of cancer.

Everyone in the study group was a member of the Seventh-day Adventist Church, a denomination that has stressed a healthy lifestyle for more than a hundred years. Because of their healthier way of life, today Adventists are one of the most researched groups in the world.

The study was a bold undertaking. Before that time, most scientific studies involved samples of 200 to 500 individuals. Rarely did they then—or even today—involve more than a thousand people. Few research projects have followed members of a comparison group for more than a decade. The enormously large sample, along with the long-term follow-up, makes the results of this study much more impressive and believable.

For twenty-three years, Jan W. Kuzma was the chairman of the Department of Biostatistics for the School of Public Health at Loma Linda University. In 1982, he became the director of research. A team of biostatisticians and epidemiologists, with Dr. Roland Phillips as primary investigator, collected, verified, followed up, analyzed, and reported the results of what is currently called the Adventist Health Study. Jan retired from the university in 1990. Dr. Gary Fraser is the current director.

We call the healthy lifestyle of these study groups the Live-Longer Lifestyle. But our information doesn't only come from this research. Studies in the Netherlands, Norway, and Poland based their work on smaller Adventist populations. Those three studies also reported that

Adventists were healthier and lived longer than the general population among whom they dwelt.

If you're wondering if this increased longevity is available only to those of the Adventist persuasion, we want to assure you that it has little to do with *being* an Adventist and everything to do with the Adventist *lifestyle*—adapting the health practices we have identified. The way we live makes the difference in our health and in our longevity.

We know firsthand the benefits of this program. Both of us have adopted the Live-Longer Lifestyle Principles.

Jan W. Kuzma, an Adventist, has followed the Live-Longer Lifestyle Principles since he was a teenager.

After Cec Murphey, a Presbyterian, had his second hospitalization with ulcers, he decided to make lifestyle changes. He weighed 25 pounds more than his present weight. His blood pressure had already reached the high normal range of 140/80, and he knew that both his parents suffered from high blood pressure.

"Congratulations. You are now going to be a chronic ulcer patient," his doctor had told him. "I'll see a lot of you after this."

But when he left the doctor's office, Cec vowed that he would never have to be treated for an ulcer again. As he prayed for guidance, he admitted he was in bad physical shape. He didn't eat right and hadn't exercised for years. During those weeks of searching for answers, he read one Bible verse that pushed him onto the pathway of change: "So, whether you eat or drink, or whatever you do, do all to the glory of God" (1 Cor. 10:31 RSV).

He realized that he regularly mistreated God's holy temple, so he began to make changes. Today, he alternates days between running and walking and averages 35 miles a week. His body is trim; his blood pressure hovers around 110/60; he hasn't needed medical attention for more than a decade.

His lifestyle change took place gradually—exactly what we advocate in this book—but it has paid off in results for him.

It has also paid off for thousands of others.

This can be your story too.

God can—and wants to—help. God wants us to live longer and healthier.

Think about that—God wants us healthier!

Ten Years Longer? Really?

Actually, the title of this book isn't quite accurate.

We're presenting the results of the Adventist Health Study. On the average, those in the program did and have lived about nine years longer than those in the control group. But here's even better news: Those who followed ALL the principles of the Live-Longer Lifestyle lived an average of thirteen years longer than their statistical life expectancy! Our research says that the closer we come to following the guidelines of the Live-Longer Lifestyle, the greater the benefit.

So why don't you prepare to live thirteen—or even more—years longer and healthier?

Most of us were born with the birthright to enjoy good health and a sense of well-being. Through our decisions, frequently influenced by our peers and the media, we choose either to maintain this birthright or to give it up.

Too often we accept the fatalistic view that it's normal to have a heart attack or stroke. *It's not normal.* We can prevent those fatal illnesses, especially those that strike in middle age.

Think carefully about having an extra decade of life—ten more years of active, healthy life. How much effort would you put into your day-to-day living if you knew it would pay off in less pain, fewer illnesses, a minimal amount of worry, and a more positive outlook on life?

Before you answer that question, we want to assure you that we're not suggesting you jump into an exercise program of jerking, bouncing, and kicking gyrations. We don't advocate a highly restrictive eating program of tasteless, boring choices. If you follow the example of the people in the Live-Longer studies, you will learn to eat healthful foods, but you will never have to give up taste or worry about portion size. *Isn't that good news?*

Here's another bit of good news about individuals who live happier lives: They don't diet. Yet fewer of them have weight problems than the general population. *They don't diet because they don't need to.* Sensible eating habits regulate their weight.

Wouldn't it be more fun to be in charge of your life? To learn to live by *principles* of good nutrition instead of slavishly following rules?

It can happen!

You can live ten more healthy, happy years.

Through this book, *you* can learn to adopt and follow a plan that will extend your years, enrich your life, and enable you to honor your body as God's holy temple. You can learn more about the food you eat, your behavior, and your attitudes. And you can learn how to relate more effectively to other human beings.

Wouldn't you like to be one of these long-living, healthier people?

God has made me responsible for my health.
I will care for my body.

HERE ARE A FEW STATISTICS FROM THE ADVENTISTS HEALTH STUDY (AHS).

AHS men lived an average of 81.9 years—9 years longer than the average California male; AHS women lived 86 years—7.5 years longer than the average California female. (And don't forget: Those who followed the Live-Longer Lifestyle lived an average of thirteen years longer than those who didn't.)

Another way to view the impressive results of following the AHS and dietary habits is to look at the four most common causes of death (aside from accidents).

Cause of Death:	Californians	AHS Subjects
Coronary heart disease	100	55
Diabetes	100	55
Bronchitis and emphysema	100	32
Lung cancer	100	20

This means that for every 100 Californians who died from coronary heart disease, only 55 of the control group died—about half the number.

GET AN ATTITUDE!

CHAPTER 2

"HIS MIND is so sick, you can't expect his body to be any better," said the elderly, uneducated woman. "Why, he frets all the time about every little thing. So how can he be healthy?" She was referring to her thirty-four-year-old neighbor, about whom she said, "That man swallows down more pills every day than I ever had in my whole life."

. . .

Despite her lack of formal education, she had a keen understanding of human nature. By observing people most of her life, she had grasped something many of us are just beginning to accept: Our mental state affects our health.

To put it another way, if you want to live ten years longer, you need to do more than consider your body. Long life also involves your thoughts and feelings. Today, most of us know that those with a fighting spirit—a positive mental attitude—have a better chance of not getting sick. And if they do become ill, they recover more quickly.

A number of studies support this:

- A British study that spanned a decade compared fifty-seven women who had undergone mastectomies. Of that group, twenty-four accepted their diagnosis and died within the decade. Those with a fighting spirit were still alive after the study ended. The work essentially compared the 40 percent who accepted their diagnosis and died to the 60 percent with a fighting spirit who survived.

- Socially active, married people tend to live longer than less-active, separated, divorced, or single people. Happily married women have the strongest immune systems. Men who participate in social activities at least once a week outlive men who don't.

- Confiding in someone else can result in a significant improvement in immune-system function.

- Men who were most pessimistic at age twenty-five had more severe illness beginning in their forties than more optimistic men of their age group.

- Pessimists are more likely to get colds than optimists are.

- Apparently, just thinking about love can raise the levels of salivary immunoglobulin A in some individuals. This is an important part of our immune system that protects us from infections and illness.

Food also affects attitude. Despite the overwhelming evidence, many still find that difficult to believe. Yet if we think about it, it seems obvious.

Food is a serious subject. Even a slight deficiency in any of thirty to forty known nutrients can change our emotional state because these nutrients affect the biochemistry and function of the brain. Small deficiencies can cause irritability, fatigue, or depression. For example: Your brain needs tryptophan to make an important transmitter called serotonin. If you eat high amounts of carbohydrates, you make it easier for your brain to draw tryptophan from the blood into the brain. If you get too much serotonin in your brain cells, you become sleepy. But you don't need to worry. Eating a wide variety of plant-based foods in as close to their original state as possible provides the safety factor in getting all essential nutrients.

In 1987, Candace Pert, at the National Institute of Mental Health, suggested that there is a molecular equivalent of telephone lines between the brain and the immune system. She said that white blood cells receive messages directly from the brain to fight off disease invaders. Attitude helps to determine the content of those messages.

Current research is proving her statements are correct.

LIVING EXAMPLES

How does this mind-body connection work in practical ways?

J. C. Penney, the genius behind one of the world's largest chains of department stores, had worked hard and built his business to a multimillion-dollar level. Then he lost forty million dollars in the stock market crash of 1929. By 1932, when he was forty-six years old, he was forced to sell out to satisfy his creditors. This left him virtually broke. He worried so much he couldn't sleep. The stress from his chronic fatigue depressed his immune system, and he suffered a relapse of the chickenpox virus that had been dormant in his body since he had had the rash as a child. (The recurrence of this virus is called shingles and causes severe pain.)

In the hospital, Penney began to recover physically. Yet he was broken mentally and overwhelmed with a fear of death. Because he didn't expect to live through the night, he wrote farewell letters to his wife and son.

The next morning, singing from the hospital chapel awakened him. Penney got out of bed, followed the music to its source, and sat down in the back of the chapel. The staff sang, "Be not dismayed, whate'er betide, God will take care of you."

He said:

I felt as if I had been instantly lifted out of the darkness of a dungeon into warm, brilliant sunlight. I felt as if I had been transported from hell to paradise. I felt the power of God as I had never felt it before. I realized that I alone was responsible for all my troubles. I knew that God with His love was there to help me. From that day to this, my life has been free from worry. I am seventy-one years old, and the most dramatic and glorious minutes of my life were those I spent in that chapel that morning.[1]

As a result of that experience, Penney rebuilt his financial empire to well over the billion-dollar mark. He lived long enough to celebrate his ninety-fifth birthday.

Attitude counts.

In recent years, we have been hearing this message from a diverse group of people who have proved it through their own lives. Dr. Bernie Siegel stresses this in his best-selling books. Louise Hay shows impressive results from teaching people to believe in and visualize success and healing. It's hard to find a top speaker on the lecture circuit who doesn't talk this language.

Those high achievers know something and have proved it by their experience.

Isn't it time for us Christians to follow God's directive about a merry heart being good for our health?

THE OPTIMIST VERSUS THE PESSIMIST

The Live-Longer Lifestyle studies show that optimism is a significant reason for healthier and longer lives. Adherents simply develop a happier, more positive attitude about life.

When things go wrong at work, pessimists tend to blame themselves for not doing a better job, for not anticipating the problem, or for not having handled all the difficulties. Optimists tend not to point the finger of blame for failure or upsets; instead they consider a variety of factors. They may say such things as, "The boss was under a lot of pressure today," or "Now I've learned, so I'll do it right the next time."

Optimists feel they are in control of their lives. If things go badly, they act quickly, seek solutions, and form new plans of action. They believe they are responsible for their health. They don't merely rely on doctors or passively follow medical advice.

Here are examples of the optimistic viewpoint in action:

Norman Cousins, editor of *Saturday Review,* wrote the best-selling *Anatomy of an Illness* in which he described his recovery from a debilitating spinal disorder. He checked into a hotel and rented comic videos, such as the Marx Brothers and the Three Stooges, and viewed reruns of everything humorous on TV from *Candid Camera* to *I Love Lucy.* He learned that ten minutes of genuine belly laughter had an anesthetic effect and would give him at least two hours of pain-free sleep. Eventually Cousins recovered, beating the 500-to-1 odds. Literally, he laughed his way to health.

The American Journal of the Medical Sciences reprinted an abstract of scientific work on laughter done by Lee S. Berk of Loma Linda University and a team of researchers. For a study on such a light subject, they began their report with this heavy statement: "Positive emotional activities have been suggested as modifiers of neuroendocrine hormones involved in the classic stress response." What their research indicated was that the "mirthful laughter" experience reduced several stress hormones in the brain.[2]

David Larson, psychiatrist and medical researcher, spent ten years at the National Institutes of Health examining the data surrounding religion and good health. In his 1992 report published in the *American Journal of Psychiatry,* he said that religious commitment—by which he meant having a relationship with God and participating in religious activities—benefited both mental and physical health. In a 1987 review by Levin and Vanderpool in *Social Science Medicine,* it was reported in twenty-two of twenty-seven studies that the more often individuals went to church, the better their health. Churchgoers face lower risks of heart disease, recover from burns and hip fractures faster, and stay out of the hospital more often than those who don't worship.

Marianne Hering, in her review of the research on the relationship between religion and health, mentions the following:

- Religious people don't tend to commit suicide as often. In fact, a strong religious commitment was the best protection against suicide.

- Those who go to church are less likely to abuse drugs.

- Those who said their religious faith was important to them were seven times less likely to have abnormal diastolic blood pressure.[3]

THE POWER OF PERCEPTION

We often hear that situations don't change our moods—but our perceptions do. "We feel the way we think" is another way of saying it. This means that if you think healthy, optimistic thoughts, you tend to feel healthy and optimistic. All your thinking has a profound effect on your physical and emotional health. If you constantly see yourself in a negative light, you can easily work yourself into a state of low self-esteem and depression. You also burden your body with heavy stress.

Whenever we think the worst outcome for a situation, our body reacts as if we were actually in such a tension-filled situation. Negative thinkers frequently suffer from stress-related physical ailments such as headaches, gastrointestinal problems, and high blood pressure.

Contrary to popular belief, we weren't born either pessimists or optimists. Our thinking patterns grow out of our experiences and environment. How we perceive any situation is an automatic response—automatic in the same way we have learned to comb our hair or brush our teeth. It's a *learned* response or habit. Someone taught us or we absorbed the attitudes of those around us—whether family members, teachers, peers, or those in the media.

We probably haven't been aware of this, yet day after day messages get pounded into us, and they become encoded in our memory. As adults, we carry on automatic thinking. Silently, we carry on conversations with ourselves, interpreting situations, condemning, arguing, or seeking to understand. We call this self-talk.

We cultivate the voices that eventually direct our actions. We can learn to rethink and to refocus our thoughts in more positive ways. One method is to develop positive self-talk.

Here are seven simple steps you can take for healthy self-talk affirmation.

1. Believe that God wants you to have a healthy mental outlook and that with God's help it is possible. Read Philippians 4:13 over and over until it becomes part of you: "I can do all things through Christ who strengthens me" (NKJV).

2. Decide what you want to change and select three or four things to focus on.

3. Write affirmations in *positive,* short, clear, specific statements, as if the changes already have occurred in your life, such as:

   - "I am healthy."
   - "I like the person I am."
   - "I am a positive person."

   Jan's wife, Kay, wrote the following self-talk statement in the flyleaf of her Bible so she can read it often: "I will not allow my self-worth to be influenced by others' perceptions of me, but by my own perceptions of whether or not I am living with integrity, being humble, knowing what to take credit for, and what is a gift from God."

4. Repeat those statements several times a day. When you say them, don't evaluate their truthfulness. You are saying, "This is what I wish to be, and I speak these words as if they have already been accomplished."

5. If you find negative thoughts intruding, refute them and continue your affirmations.

6. Make these affirmations an ongoing part of your life. Spend a few minutes several times a day thoughtfully repeating your affirmations to yourself.

7. Thank God for the miracle of transformation that is taking place in your life.

THE POWER OF VISUALIZATION

The late Norman Vincent Peale in his book *How to Make Positive Imaging Work for You* wrote about being in Hong Kong and speaking to the owner of a tattoo shop. One of the designs read: "Born to Lose." Peale asked the man why anyone would want to have those words permanently imprinted on him- or herself.

"Before tattoo on chest, tattoo on mind," the man said.[4]

By contrast, many athletes have learned to *visualize their achievements*—scoring the winning run, laying the ball in the hoop, making the crucial touchdown. It's not a dreamy hope-I-can-do-it attitude. They visualize their achievements and keep those images before themselves. Often they say words of self-affirmation as well, such as, "I am at my physical peak." "I hit a home run." "I catch every fly that comes my way."

Stan Cottrell, now in his early fifties, has run more recorded miles than anyone else in the world. He ran 2,000 miles along the Great Wall of China. At one time he held the record for running from New York to San Francisco as well as having run the most miles in a twenty-four-hour period. He still runs 40 miles a day, whether it's up the Andes, across Vietnam or Europe, or around the island of the Dominican Republic.

Stan visualizes himself running vast distances. People tell him that it's physically impossible to do what he does, and then they watch him in action. He believes that anything he (or anyone else) can visualize and believe in is possible, if it is within God's will.

Achievement through visualization is not a lift-yourself-up-by-your-own-bootstraps philosophy. Rather, it's believing that God created us in the divine image and that we're the temple God wants to live in.

Our power to control and reshape our attitudes and emotions serves a double purpose: to enhance our happiness and improve our health. It comes down to this: Positive people *are* healthier.

We can better resist stress and ward off cardiovascular disease and gastrointestinal troubles. Our immune systems are less likely to break down and may even work harder to protect us against allergies, arthritis, and cancer. Our brains manufacture natural pain-relieving chemicals, so we feel better. When we do get sick, those natural painkillers often dramatically alter the course of the disease.

God has put us in charge of our lives *and our physical health*. We can control our thoughts. If we think negative thoughts, bad things are more likely to happen. Our thinking results in what some call self-fulfilling prophecy. When we think about and visualize ourselves losing weight, toning muscles, and getting well, the chances are greater that these things will happen. If we expect the good things to happen and act positively, we interact better with others and tend to find solutions to problems.

Part of the positive attitude includes belief in God, the greater power—a certainty that God cares about us and our needs. We have the privilege of laying our worries in God's hands and asking for guidance and forgiveness. We don't have to live with guilt, regret, or bitterness.

Those of us who adopt the Live-Longer Lifestyle and practice the health principles, including the power of positive thinking, learn to overcome problems. Some describe this transformation as similar to awakening from a trance. For the first time in many years, they find themselves really living and enjoying the abundant life.

THINK ABOUT SUCH THINGS

The following directions sound simple—and they are. But they will help you develop a healthier, more optimistic attitude.

1. *Smile often. Laugh a lot.* Practice thinking pleasant thoughts. Learn not to take yourself too seriously. Remind yourself that it's all right to enjoy your life. Read a joke book. Share funny stories. Aim for at least five to ten minutes of good laughter each day.

2. *When you face problems, tell yourself, "This will pass."* Most situations that upset you are often relatively insignificant. One woman learned to push past these problems by saying to herself, "Five years from now I won't even remember this incident."

   When bad things happen, it's depressing to think you might have to put up with negative conditions for a lifetime. Instead, focus on getting through one day at a time. That's all we're asked to endure. Then balance this with your hope that things will get better. Hope is a welcome companion!

3. *Develop a support network* of family members, friends, or church groups. With their help, learn to enjoy life. Ask them to help you become involved in activities.

4. *Condition your mind.* Memorize powerful Bible verses or inspirational poetry. The Bible and other positive books can help you achieve peace. Here are Jan's favorite verses: Psalms 34:1, 9, 14, 19–20; 37:4–5; 50:15; 57:10; 91:15; 103:1–2.

5. *Learn to forgive.* Pray for your enemies. As you learn to forgive those who have hurt you (intentionally or inadvertently), you learn the freedom this gives and the ensuing peace of mind.

6. *Learn to experience the power of love*—the universal source that has inspired people to do incredible things. The love Shah Jahan had for his wife drove him to spend his life and his fortune building the Taj Mahal in her memory.

Poet Elizabeth Barrett, best known for "How Do I Love Thee?" was an invalid because of a childhood accident and was confined to the house of a domineering father. When she found love in the person of the poet Robert Browning, he rescued her from an atmosphere of parental control and took her from England to Italy. There her health improved so much that she gave birth to a son. Love has tremendous potential for improving health.

7. *Think of yourself as a child of God.* The Bible provides an abundance of promises to God's children:

   - ". . . If God is for us, who can be against us?" (Rom. 8:31 NIV).

   - ". . . the one who is in you is greater than the one who is in the world" (1 John 4:4 NIV).

   - "Therefore, there is now no condemnation for those who are in Christ Jesus" (Rom. 8:1 NIV).

   - ". . . whatever you ask for in prayer, believe that you have received it, and it will be yours" (Mark 11:24 NIV).

8. *Break your negative-thinking habit.* Decide you will make every effort to think optimistically for a twenty-one-day trial period. During those three weeks, count your blessings several times each day. When you start to focus on bad situations, visualize what you want to achieve and review your positive self-talk affirmations.

9. *Think of yourself as being more than your body.* You are also your thoughts and emotions. If you focus on your body, you probably tend to view good health as an end in itself and encumber yourself with doing all the right things. An obsession with your body can cause you to be dogmatic and terribly correct in health matters and, more than likely, miserable to live with. Think of your healthy body as a means to achieving a positive, fulfilled, and abundant life. Don't let fitness rule your life and steal time away from God, family, or necessary activities.

Attitude does count. We need to aspire to be a fit temple for God, believe we can, and discover the self-fulfilling prophecy that with God's help *we become that which we believe.*

_____

*Because I choose to live longer and healthier,
I choose to think healthy thoughts.*

EATING TO LIVE

REMEMBER THE first car you ever owned? No matter what its age, to you it was probably the most beautiful piece of engineering you ever saw. You loved its reliability and the way it performed. You hoped it would last a lifetime. But after a few months, you got used to the vehicle, and occasionally you neglected its proper maintenance, such as changing the oil, replacing belts, checking the transmission, or rotating the tires.

...

Then you noticed ads touting the power of additives to improve your car's performance. You bought them, and they helped—but the effects weren't permanent. Or perhaps one additive worked against something else in the engine. In time, those small, seemingly inconsequential choices took their toll. Your car's zip disappeared, and it began to make disturbing noises under the hood. (If you were honest with yourself, you knew that most of the problems were your fault.) So you traded your vehicle for a newer one.

This parallels the way you probably treat your body. If you're like most people, you enter life robust and ready for growth, but you tend to take your body for granted and fail to think much about caring for it—until you get sick.

Does this sound familiar?

But the parallel with the car stops here because you can't trade in your body for a new one. You're stuck with the original model. The good news is that you can probably correct the major defects if you don't wait too long and if you give yourself proper care.

Health is our precious birthright, but it comes with the responsibility to care for ourselves during our entire life. That's why we should eat to live, not live to eat. We'll then increase our chances of living better while living longer.

By following the Live-Longer Lifestyle, *we will be able to enjoy our quality of life.*

LIVE AND LET LIVE?

Cec Murphey overheard this conversation between two of his friends at a sporting event. Here's a shortened version:

"Every time you turn around, somebody is telling you this or that causes cancer," Gene said as he munched on his double cheeseburger, which he had enhanced with extra mayonnaise and catsup. "We all gotta die some time, right?"

"But you may die sooner than you need to," Mike said. "Maybe you ought to be a little more concerned about the way you eat—"

"Oh, I'm concerned, all right," Gene said with a laugh. "I make sure I get plenty of food."

Later on, Gene ate two foot-long hot dogs. Mike tried again to talk about nutrition and health. Gene was already taking medication for high blood pressure, and his doctor had repeatedly urged him to cut down on his salt intake. His recent cholesterol test had revealed a dangerously high level of 330.

"Yeah, maybe," he said, "but this tastes so good. If I have to die, this is sure a fun way to go."

"In twenty years, tell me how you're feeling and let me know if it's still fun," Mike said. "That is, if you're still around."

"Hey, guy, lighten up," Gene said. "Live and let live, huh? Why spoil things for me?"

Mike's words sounded a little strong perhaps, and maybe they weren't very tactful, but he spoke out of concern for the health of his friend. Gene's attitude and responses aren't unusual.

Like Gene, many of us are tired of experts and the media telling us what foods to give up. We're bored with all the low-fat ads and angry at the latest information about what's carcinogenic. We're also tired of all the conflicting information. Some of us think "eating right" means sticking to boring foods, such as two pieces of lettuce and six carrot sticks every day for lunch. Or we're fed up with the cancer scares that regularly appear in the media.

"Why, if I listened to everybody and gave up everything bad for my health," one housewife said, "I'd starve to death."

It's not that bad, but the matter of eating *is* significant. A lot of information gets thrown into the public arena. Advertisers, more concerned about profit than nutrition, give vague or confusing information. Consumers often can't distinguish truth from the gimmicks of Madison Avenue.

So maybe good health is like the car that's performing well. When it's running smoothly, we think little about maintenance. "After all," we say in our own defense, "everything works." But if the engine blows up and we get stranded on the expressway, the experience forces us to consider seriously what we should have been doing all along to keep our car operating at maximum efficiency.

Let's apply that to our bodies and start with nutrition. If much of maintaining good health revolves around an eating lifestyle, doesn't it make sense to emphasize good nutrition?

One of the problems involved in teaching nutrition is that it doesn't have an immediate cause-and-effect result. Our bodies can withstand a lot of mistreatment. They can endure despite all the junk food and poisons we ingest. That is, for a period of time. But eventually such mistreatment catches up with us.

EATING THE RIGHT KINDS OF FOOD

To start making good, healthful choices, we need to understand the reason for eating the right kinds of food.

First, food forms all the cells and tissues of our bodies. Perception, memory, and all the intricate complexities are possible because our bodies have enzymes, hormones, genes, and thousands of other wonders produced *through the food we eat*. Our bodies aren't static like the statue in the local park. Our cells die and need to be replaced. Molecular units within our cells shift constantly.

Food is responsible for body structure. Even more amazing is that we don't have a single body molecule or chemical that we had seven years ago. In just seven years, each of us has an almost total body replacement.

What we eat and how our bodies handle the food is the miracle that makes this happen. Because that's true—and provable—doesn't it make sense to choose carefully what we eat?

Second, food is our bodies' energy source. When combined with oxygen, food provides us with energy.

Energy comes from three types of food: carbohydrates, fats, and proteins. In a general way, carbohydrates (starches and sugars) are used as immediate energy; fats are high-energy storage; proteins are the body building blocks. But their roles also overlap. Our bodies can use protein and fat for energy, or they can convert excess glucose (sugar) to either fat or glycogen (animal starch).

To complicate this, proteins and carbohydrates have the same caloric value, 4 calories to a gram. (A teaspoon of liquid is approximately 5 grams.) However, fats have more than twice the energy value—9 calories to a gram.

Our bodies "burn" food.

Calorie refers to the amount of heat needed to raise the temperature of one liter of water 1°C at sea level. More simply, if you're average, you have to burn 3,500 calories to lose one pound of weight.

To stay alive, we need a minimum number of calories. The amount varies among individuals—somewhere from 1,000 to 1,700 daily to maintain brain function, circulation, respiration, and digestion. Our activity levels determine how many calories we need to go about the normal activities of life. As a general rule, women need 2,000 calories a day, and men need about 2,700.

MAKING THE MOST OF FOOD

You can use food to the maximum if you follow a few simple rules.

1. *Eat slowly and enjoy your food.* When you're feeling pressured, your overloaded system doesn't handle digestion properly.

    Some complain that they don't have time to eat leisurely meals. That's reason enough to relax and eat slowly. If you have only a limited amount of time, it's better to eat less than to gulp down your food.

Here's a diet tip:

People who eat slowly tend to eat less. It's one way to limit the quantity of food. The more you eat, the more the digestive system has to work.

2. *Chew thoroughly.* The digestive process begins in the mouth, not the stomach. By chewing your food longer, you prepare your food with more salivary amylase (enzymes needed for better processing in the stomach—a kind of predigesting process).

Ponder this general rule:

The closer to the natural state, the more nutritious the food—and the more you will need to chew. Those who eat a lot of raw and unprocessed foods enjoy better health.

3. *Limit the variety of food you eat at each meal.* Keep it simple. Three or four separate dishes are enough variety for most people.

> **Try this:**
> Don't make a habit of serving food in courses. It's easy to overeat if you don't realize how much is yet to come.

4. *Enjoy moderate exercise after meals.* Many of us can remember eating a heavy lunch and having to sit in a classroom or meeting. Our minds may have felt dull for an hour or so. We may even have fallen asleep. Too much food dulls mental activity and blunts the memory and perceptive faculties.

5. *Avoid eating immediately after heavy exertion.* Digestion demands more from your system than most of us realize. Heavy exercise just before a meal may prevent your digestive organs from getting the resources they need. It is better if you can allow a little time to relax before eating.

6. *Space meals five or six hours apart.* Don't eat until your stomach has had a chance to rest from the hard labor of digesting the previous meal. Those of us who have trouble spacing our eating have learned to drink a lot of water between meals. Not only is it healthful, but drinking one or two glasses of water can also fool our bodies into thinking we're not hungry. This makes the stomach feel full without adding calories to digest.

7. *Consider eating two meals a day.* Some have found this works best for shedding pounds. Others, as they grow older, see eliminating one meal as a way to prevent weight gain. It's not the lifestyle for everyone.

   When most people decide to eat only two meals a day, they usually cut breakfast. But that's the one meal *not* to avoid. In fact, make breakfast the *largest* meal of the day. Your body needs more food at the start of the work day than at the end. The meal to skip is in the evening.

8. *Eat meals at regular hours.* Our bodies readily adapt to cycles and rhythms, and they function best when events such as meals come at regular, fixed times each day. Initially, some people experience discomfort in making this change, but our bodies adjust after a few attempts.

If I make wise, informed choices about my eating,
I can expect to live ten healthy years longer.

EATING SECRETS

CHAPTER 4

"YOU MEAN if I follow these eating suggestions," Richard Clark asks, "they'll add years to my life?"

. . .

"Probably, Richard," we say. "But even more important, you'll be healthier and able to enjoy your life a lot more."

"And it's that simple?" he asks, his skepticism obvious in his voice.

"That's right. Follow these simple guidelines. We call them secrets only because few people seem aware of them or are willing to put in the effort to add years of health and vitality."

Richard, still unsure, says, "I'm open to listening."

That's all we ask. Here are eleven eating secrets practiced by those who follow the Live-Longer Lifestyle that can dramatically change your life.

SECRET 1: THEY EAT A PLANT-BASED DIET

This is the single, major dietary secret of those who follow the Live-Longer Lifestyle: *They are vegetarians.* That fact, above everything else, accounts for their better health.

Although we have both chosen to be vegetarians, we realize that most people won't follow our lifestyle. It *is* a choice. Our purpose here is to

29

present maximum health benefits. Eliminating meat, for instance, is a step in the right direction. Each step toward the nonuse of meat, fish, and poultry presents the opportunity for better health and longer life.

"Vegetarianism? You mean I have to give up meat?" That's often the first response we get.

But that's not the right question to ask. It's not a matter of giving up something; it's a matter of shifting to a healthier lifestyle. The healthiest individuals choose not to eat meat. It is a deliberate choice. It's not based on deprivation ("I can't eat meat") but on a decision to opt for better nutrition ("I can eat anything I want; I choose not to eat meat").

Although some people in the ongoing study are meat-eaters (which includes fish and poultry), they eat only the "clean" meats according to Leviticus 11. Those who follow the complete Live-Longer Lifestyle do not ingest any form of meat. In addition, many have either given up dairy products and eggs or have greatly reduced their intake as more information has become available concerning the harmful effects of high cholesterol and the potential diseases found in animal products.

Regardless of the kind of food you grew up with or have grown accustomed to, it is possible to train your taste buds and your attitudes so that you won't desire meat. If you value health, wouldn't it be foolish not to explore ways to eat that will enhance that health? ways that will give you more energy? ways that will keep you free from disease and sickness?

What Is a Vegetarian?

Some people who don't eat red meat but do eat chicken and fish call themselves vegetarians. Strictly speaking, they aren't. Two lighthearted statements that vegetarians use to make their point are, "I don't eat anything that ever had a mother" and "I don't eat anything that ever had a face."

There are two kinds of vegetarians. *Most are lacto-ovo vegetarians*—they eat some animal products, such as eggs, cheese, yogurt, and milk, but usually in small amounts. *Vegans* eat and use only plant products.

The Live-Longer Lifestyle studies indicate significant findings about the vegetarians they studied:

1. They are better educated than the average American citizen.

2. They exercise more.

3. Fewer are overweight.

4. Fewer had the flu or a cold during the previous year.

5. They pay attention to the *way* they eat. We need food for energy and body structure, but food is also something to enjoy. The Live-Longer Lifestyle studies show that those who have combined good health with longevity actually enjoy good eating. They sometimes speak of learning to savor their food. For them, the aroma and flavor are integral parts of eating. Too often, people learn to use food to assuage feelings of loneliness, sadness, guilt, or anger.

Why would anyone want to become a vegetarian? Jan has heard that question a thousand times. He answers it this way: "First, it's a healthier lifestyle—it decreases our chances of developing illnesses; helps us live more healthy, pain-free lives; and, consequently, adds years to our lives. Second, this lifestyle increases our physical stamina. More and more sports enthusiasts are becoming living examples of this."

Although Jan has been a vegetarian since he was a teenager, he knows that most people don't choose to make a drastic shift to vegetarianism. He encourages those who want to live longer and healthier to make one change at a time, moving slowly toward their ultimate goal. He also suggests simple steps, such as substituting poultry for red meat and increasing the intake of plant foods. Eventually their taste for meat will disappear, and they'll feel better.

"I understand that part," Carol Clark says, "but can I get enough protein as a vegetarian? We have to have protein, don't we?"

True, your body needs protein, but it doesn't have to come from animal sources.

That fact surprised Carol—and many others. Most people assume protein (which is made up of amino acids) comes only from meat and dairy products. Most Americans also eat more animal protein than they need. The average consumption is in excess of 100 grams every day (about four ounces of meat). While individuals' needs vary, a medium-sized man requires only 63 grams and a medium-sized woman about 46 grams.

Can Vegetarians Get Enough Protein?

In the 1980s it became popular to speak of "complete proteins" or "complementary proteins"—a combination of at least two foods, such as rice and beans, to form a whole protein. This was standard thinking based on experiments conducted between 1929 and 1950. More recent studies, however, show that eating a variety of foods provides the body with all the needed amino acids—the source for making complete protein for our daily needs.

A healthy diet doesn't need a lot of protein—less than 15 percent of your food intake is sufficient. If you eat a wide variety of fruit, vegetables, and grains, you don't have to worry about protein deficiency.

Here are the major arguments that support the vegetarian lifestyle.

1. *You don't have to eat meat to get necessary vitamins.* Plants provide eleven of the thirteen needed vitamins. The two missing are

vitamin D and vitamin B₁₂. Your body produces vitamin D when you're exposed to sunlight. The bacteria in your intestines makes vitamin B₁₂ (or you can supplement with brewer's yeast, fortified soy milk, or over-the-counter supplements). That's all you need.

2. *You can get all the minerals you need by eating a variety of unprocessed, natural foods.* All minerals originate in the ground. Plants absorb and store them.

3. *Vegetables are high in fiber—which meat lacks.* Fiber is essential for maintaining proper bowel function, stabilizing blood sugar levels, and removing excess cholesterol.

4. *The high concentration of protein in meat causes an overwhelming loss of the body's calcium through the kidneys.* This can result in osteoporosis. The purines in meat become uric acid and can also cause gout and kidney stones.

5. *Improperly cooked meats can cause diseases* such as cancer, hepatitis, salmonella, staphylococcus, trichinosis, and toxoplasmosis. And it's sometimes difficult to know if meat has been cooked thoroughly.

6. *Meat may contain unhealthy substances.* Animals ingest *and store* chemicals in their muscles and tissues from fertilizers and pesticides used on their food. Random samples show that meat frequently contains residues of antibiotics and hormones the animals received before slaughter. Although we have laws to protect against this, much of the retail meat doesn't actually get checked.

7. *Statistically, vegetarians are slimmer, healthier, and longer lived* than the average person. This is confirmed not only by the Live-Longer Lifestyle studies but also by studies of other groups, such as Mormons, who tend to eat less meat than average Americans.

8. *Some vegetarians argue that the body is designed for plant foods.* Humans have hands instead of claws. Our teeth grind instead of rip. (Meat-eating animals swallow in gulps without chewing because they have no molars; their stomachs contain a strong acid to break

down fibrous tissues and bones.) Humans also have long intestines designed to digest plant parts.

The human body can nourish itself on both plant and animal food if necessary, but wouldn't it be better to fuel it with the plant-based foods it was designed for?

"Hey, wait a minute," says the voice of protest. "What about Eskimos? They don't eat vegetables; they live on nothing but fat and meat!"

That's right, or at least it has been with traditional Eskimos, who lead the world in per capita consumption of meat and fat. What most people don't know is that Eskimos

- age rapidly
- have high rates of disease
- have an *average* life span of only thirty-five to forty years

The saving factor in their diet is a high intake of omega-3 oil, which is important for balancing the negative aspects of other oils.

By contrast, the Hunza from the mountains near India commonly live eighty-five to one hundred years. These vegetarians farm the hillsides and eat the food they grow. They have almost no disease and stay active and fit throughout their lifetimes.

Here's a fact to think about:
The highest occurrences of heart disease, cancer, and diabetes occur in the nations that consume the most meat.

Protein Misconceptions
Americans have heard so much about getting enough protein that a variety of untruths have become accepted. Here are eight commonly believed fallacies about protein.

1. "We need a lot of protein every day for good health." Fact: Our bodies use protein efficiently—a little goes a long way.

2. "Athletes need extra protein for strength and endurance." Fact: Research doesn't agree. High-protein diets and even protein supplements touted by athletes are expensive and stressful to the body. Strive for a balanced diet.

3. "We need a lot of red meat because it builds muscle." Fact: Meat protein doesn't go directly to the muscles. Our bodies process it the same way they do all food.

4. "Protein foods are low in calories and good for dieters." Fact: Actually, proteins have the same number of calories as carbohydrates—4 for each gram. Many proteins, such as beef, are *high in fat,* which has 9 calories per gram.

5. "A high-protein diet is the best way to lose weight." Fact: Proteins can't burn fat, as some people have claimed. High-protein diets aren't balanced and can strain the kidneys. Liquid protein diets can be dangerous, especially to the heart.

6. "Protein will provide extra energy." Fact: Carbohydrates are the body's most efficient energy source.

7. "Vegetables don't have any protein." Fact: Most vegetables contain some protein. By eating a wide variety of vegetables each day, most people should have no concern about getting enough protein.

8. "Older people don't need protein because they're no longer growing." Fact: While it's true that infants and children need the most protein for each pound of body weight, everyone needs some protein each day for good health. Experts recommend 12 to 15 percent of a healthful diet be protein food.

SECRET 2: THEY HAVE REDUCED OR ELIMINATED THEIR CONSUMPTION OF DAIRY PRODUCTS

When you were in school, didn't you learn that milk was the perfect food? You were told that milk makes muscles big, teeth strong, and your body beautiful. This information came from the National Dairy Council.

Today, many nutrition-minded people feel that healthy eating includes cutting back or even eliminating milk. Nutritional experts stand divided into two groups: those against the use of dairy products and those who see no problem with them.

One of the main arguments for using dairy products is our need for calcium. However, many green and yellow vegetables, as well as fruits, give plentiful amounts of calcium. People who regularly eat broccoli, grains, beans, and nuts, for example, get all the calcium their bodies require.

There are several good reasons to cut back—way back—on dairy products.

1. *Most adults don't have the digestive equipment to use milk efficiently.* Around age four, most people lose the ability to produce two enzymes: rennin and lactase. Rennin breaks down the protein of cow's milk; lactase breaks down lactose, the natural sugar in milk.

    In spite of this lack, we live in a culture that continues to insist we must have what comes from dairy cows for good nutrition. Americans use 75 billion pounds of dairy products every year. That comes out to roughly 300 pounds for every person in the nation.

2. *Dairy products are now being implicated in a variety of food allergies.* Milk product allergies can cause:

    - gastrointestinal problems: canker sores, vomiting, colic, stomach cramps, colitis, loss of appetite, diarrhea, constipation, or painful defecation
    - respiratory problems: hay fever, asthma, bronchitis, sinusitis, colds, runny noses, or ear infections (all possibly due to increased mucus production)

- skin problems: rashes, atopic dermatitis, eczema, seborrhea, or hives
- behavioral problems: irritability, restlessness, hyperactivity, headache, lethargy, fatigue, muscle pain, or depression
- other potential problems: migraine headaches or iron deficiency anemia

3. *Dairy products contain cholesterol and saturated fats,* just like meat. Some nutritionists call milk "liquid meat."

4. *Dairy products can contribute to the onset of osteoporosis* because they are high in protein. High-protein diets rob your body of calcium. Despite the aggressive campaigning by the National Dairy Council, reputable researchers state that even though milk is high in calcium, the more you drink, the more calcium you lose.

"Wisconsin is the number one osteoporosis state, and it is the number one dairy state," says Dr. John Reinhold, executive director of the Medi-Share Program. "Scandinavia and other high dairy-consuming nations all have the highest levels of osteoporosis."

Harvard University researchers studied 77,761 women, ages thirty-four to fifty-nine, over a twelve-year period. They reported a greater risk for osteoporitic hip and forearm fractures in women who drank two or more glasses of milk daily. They compared their sample with women of the same age group who consumed no more than one glass a week.

Many health-conscious individuals have turned to substitutes—milklike products made from soy or rice. Most supermarkets now carry such products.

More recently, however, Dr. Dean Ornish and other leaders in the field of nutrition are allowing people to use "blue" or skim milk.

If you're using whole milk and want to switch to skim milk, you'll probably find the taste and texture change easier to get

used to if you substitute 2 percent for whole milk first. Then use
1 percent for a while before switching to skim.

SECRET 3: THEY REGULARLY EAT BREAKFAST

Emphasis on breakfast often surprises dieters, but the truly health-
minded consider it the most important meal of the day. The theory is that
the body needs more food at the start of the workday than at the end.
Eating the bulk of our daily calories in the evening can lead to obesity.

People function at their best when they start the day with a good
meal. The famous Iowa Breakfast Studies (conducted from 1949 to
1961) were the first to focus attention on the effects of eating breakfast. They concluded that adults who ate breakfast could perform
physical and mental tasks in the late morning more efficiently with
faster reaction times and less neuromuscular tremor than those who
skipped the morning meal.

SECRET 4: THEY EAT MORE FRESH VEGETABLES

A healthy lifestyle requires plenty of vegetables. Here are six significant reasons to eat your vegetables.

1. *Vegetables are high in vitamins and minerals.* Did you know that
   some vegetables contain more calcium than milk? They are broccoli, kale, collards, mustard greens, turnip greens, dandelion
   greens, parsley, watercress, and kelp (a sea vegetable).

2. *Vegetables are excellent sources of dietary fiber.* Without fiber, sometimes called the "intestinal broom," toxic wastes build up in your
   system and gradually poison your entire body. Lack of dietary
   fiber can cause a number of illnesses, including chronic constipation, gas, bloating, diverticulosis, and chronic fatigue.

   Consuming adequate dietary fiber also helps you lose weight.

Fiber, once called "roughage," is the part of fruits, vegetables, and grains that your body can't digest. Fiber passes through your system whole, which has caused some to call it weight management's best friend.

Eating a variety of high-fiber foods helps keep the colon functioning properly. Many health professionals consider a poorly functioning colon a fundamental cause of degenerative disease. The British Medical Society has even stated that "death begins in the colon."

3. *Vegetables contain anticancer nutrients.* Veggies high in beta carotene (a plant form of vitamin A) together with phytochemicals wage war against cancer. Carrots, cabbage, broccoli, Brussels sprouts, kohlrabi, cauliflower, and yams (or sweet potatoes) do the best job.

4. *Vegetables are low in fat and have no cholesterol.*

5. *Vegetables are safer to eat than meat.* They are low on the food chain, which means they contain lower levels of contaminants from pesticides and other environmental toxins than farm animals, who store concentrated amounts of pollutants in their flesh and fat.

6. *Raw vegetables are loaded with health-producing nutrients, especially enzymes.* Cooking begins to destroy enzymes at 107°F and completely destroys them at 122°F; microwaving destroys all enzymes. If you're not eating a wide variety of non-cooked foods, we suggest you try nutritional supplements.

SECRET 5: THEY EAT MORE FRESH FRUIT THAN AVERAGE AMERICANS

For maximum benefit, we need to eat at least six servings of fruit a day. Here are three important reasons for eating plenty of fresh fruit.

1. *Fruit is cleansing.* Most are about 90 percent liquid. Fruit juice is a health-promoting fluid that helps clean out your system by flushing your cells, bathing your tissues, and stimulating the workings of your metabolic processes. Fruit also contains dietary fiber.

2. *Fruit provides satisfaction.* Fruit satisfies your desire for sweets in a healthful, natural way. But even more important, fruit contains all the necessary ingredients for your body to sustain life, including glucose from carbohydrates for energy, vitamins, minerals, fatty acids, and amino acids for the building of protein.

3. *Fruit delivers energy.* No bodily function requires more energy than the digestion of food. The natural sugars in fruit give your body an energy boost while demanding virtually no digestive energies from you. Ripe fruit and fresh juices (not bottled or frozen) are loaded with their own digestive enzymes that go to work quickly in the stomach. It takes only about thirty minutes for fruit to release nutrients into the intestines for absorption.

Drying fruit preserves nutrients better than freezing or cooking. One dried fruit that often gets overlooked is the fig. Dr. Samuel DeShay, in his book, *Plus Fifteen,* calls the fig nature's most nearly perfect fruit. It has a high dietary fiber content, unequaled by other common fresh and dried fruits. The fig has the highest overall mineral content found in common fruit, and it contains the calcium and magnesium needed to keep bones and teeth strong while helping to lower blood pressure. Potassium, also found in figs, is essential to heartbeat regulation, nerve transmission, and metabolism.

You might also want to try dates, raisins, and prunes. They're also high in potassium and vitamin A, as are watermelon, cantaloupe, peaches, apricots, and avocados.

SECRET 6: THEY EAT MORE GRAINS AND NUTS

Nutritionists have long stressed the importance of whole-grain bread. But don't limit your bread to whole wheat flour; enjoy a variety of grains.

Bread is only one way to use grains and nuts. Whole grains also make great breakfast foods and entrees. They are simple to cook, especially if you have a Crockpot. Put a cup of grain, such as whole wheat, barley, corn, millet, or oats, and plenty of water in your Crockpot before you go to bed and the next morning you'll have perfectly cooked grain for the day.

Nuts need little in the way of preparation. Most of them—for example, walnuts and almonds—can be eaten raw. Nuts are unusual among natural vegetable foods. Although 80 percent of their calories come from fat, it's beneficial fat, as most contain monounsaturated fat. Walnuts, however, have a high amount of polyunsaturated fat. Nuts are also an excellent source of dietary fiber, vitamin E—which protects against heart disease—and omega-3 oils. Cooking with nuts as part of a main entree provides high-quality protein low in saturated fat.

One warning about nuts: Since they are high in fat, they are also high in calories. That's why you should eat them in limited quantities. If you have difficulty controlling your nut intake, buy them in their natural state—in the shell. That should slow your eating down considerably!

SECRET 7: THEY EAT MORE LEGUMES

Legumes are plants that have seeds growing inside pods; this classification includes beans and lentils. Not only are legumes a simple substitute for meat, but they also

- are inexpensive and easily prepared.

- can be mixed and flavored in countless ways to provide nutritious and filling entrees or side dishes.
- are an important source of fiber.
- lower cholesterol.
- contain fewer calories than meat. (One cup of beans has only 250 calories compared to 550 in five ounces of steak.)
- are an excellent source of protein and carbohydrates. (Most legumes are 20 to 30 percent protein.)

If you want to improve the quality of your diet by reducing or eliminating meat and dairy products—which will lower your LDL or "bad" cholesterol—legumes are the best replacement. You can incorporate this neglected food group into your diet in the form of any of the two dozen varieties available, including split peas, black-eyed peas, or a variety of beans, such as kidney, lima, navy, garbanzos (chickpeas), soy, and black.

SECRET 8: THEY HAVE REDUCED THEIR FAT INTAKE AND USE UNREFINED OILS

While you need some fat in your diet, the Live-Longer Lifestyle recommends that fat should be less than 20 percent of your daily caloric intake. Most experts, however, consider 30 percent as a more realistic figure. If you're an average American, 37 percent of your daily calories come from fat—definitely not low enough to protect you from heart disease.

Fat—concentrated energy—provides you with essential fatty acids, helps you to absorb fat-soluble vitamins, adds flavor to your food, and gives you a feeling of satisfaction when you have finished eating.

Your body can't make those necessary fatty acids, so you have to eat them. However, you can get them from plant sources. Your body converts fatty acids into substances that regulate many body processes, including normal cell growth and activity and proper nerve function. The substances made from these essential fatty acids also help you maintain hormonal balance to lower your blood pressure and cholesterol count, decrease the clumping of blood cells, and resist various diseases.

Although typical Western diets contain too much fat, too little can result in caloric deficiency, dry skin, decreased resistance to disease, irregular or lack of menses, muscle atrophy, and retarded growth in children.

Because *fat* and *cholesterol* are two words that bring confusion and misunderstanding, we have devoted chapter 10 to just this issue.

SECRET 9: THEY HAVE REDUCED THEIR USE OF REFINED FOODS, ESPECIALLY SUGAR

The refining process tends to concentrate the valueless components in food, which adds more calories and subtracts nutrition. Let's look at two examples.

First we'll examine the apple. A delicious apple with its natural sweetness contains about 70 calories. When refined and concentrated into a cup of apple juice, the calories increase to 120. Refine that same apple into a slice of apple pie, and the number zooms to 350.

Second, consider the potato. A plain, baked potato has about 100 calories. When made into French fries, the calories soar to 300. Hash browns soaked in animal fat have no trouble coming in at 400 calories. When that same potato gets turned into chips, the calories are a staggering 800.

Refined sugar has no vitamins. It contains no minerals. In spite of its lack of benefit, most Americans eat between 120 and 150 pounds of refined sugar annually. Some refer to sugar as empty energy.

Sugar: Empty Energy

Refined sugar is more than empty calories. This prolific food ingredient can actually harm the body.

1. Your body rapidly absorbs refined sugar into the bloodstream, which produces a rise in blood sugar levels and makes the pancreas excrete large amounts of insulin. This can cause a rapid drop in blood sugar, resulting in hypoglycemic or low blood sugar symptoms.

2. Refined sugar can irritate the gastrointestinal tract as it breaks down to glucose and fructose.

3. Your body must have vitamin B_1 to process sugar. Too much sugar can cause a vitamin B_1 deficiency.

4. Sugar isn't filling, which makes it easier to eat excessive amounts. This often results in weight gain.

5. A high consumption of refined sugar can predispose you to diabetes.

6. Refined sugar can increase your LDL (bad) cholesterol level.

7. Refined sugar causes cavities in your teeth.

8. Refined sugar interferes with your white blood cells' ability to fight infections. (The effect can last for several hours.)

If you are typical, you use more than a third of a pound of sugar a day—600 calories of health-destroying sweetness. The results show up in an epidemic of tooth decay, weight problems, diabetes, and other diseases that scientists are beginning to link to high sugar consumption.

"Awful, but I don't have a sweet tooth," you say, "so I'm safe from all that sugar."

Think again!

More than two-thirds of the refined sugar we eat is "hidden sugar," sugar that has been added to manufactured products. Did you know that manufacturers put sugar in salt? And did you know that a tablespoon of regular catsup contains a teaspoon of refined sugar?

If that surprises you, consider these popular food items that are laced with sugar: peanut butter, pickles, canned fruits and vegetables, mayonnaise, bread, many juices, soup, cereal, cured meat, hot dogs, lunch meat, salad dressings, spaghetti sauce, crackers, tomato juice, and pasta products.

Even people who are careful to read labels often don't realize how much sugar they're actually getting. The reason: Sugar comes in a variety of forms, and manufacturers often combine several in a single product.

The answer is moderation—limit the amount of all kinds of sugar in your diet.

What Kind of Sugar?

Manufacturers use a number of types of hidden sugars in their products. Here are the different terms for sugar you'll find on labels.

Sucrose, commonly known as refined white table sugar, comes from sugar cane, sugar beets, and sugar maples. It's the most widely used form of sugar, but it can also cause the most health problems because it demands the production of insulin by your pancreas. This creates significant fluctuation in blood sugar levels and robs nutrients from various stores in your body.

A popular misconception is that candy and other sweets high in sucrose will provide "quick energy." Although they will give you a temporary "sugar high," this high also precedes the "sugar blues." As the old saying goes, "What goes up, must come down."

Fructose (also known as *levulose*) occurs naturally in fruits and honey, or it can be commercially refined from corn, sugar beets, and sugar cane. Corn syrup is the most common form, and refined fructose is about 70 percent sweeter than sucrose.

Maltose comes from "malting" certain grains together with natural enzymes. Two of the most popular forms are barley malt and brown rice syrup.

Glucose (also known as *dextrose*) appears naturally in fruit, honey, carob, and corn or in its refined form. It's about two-thirds as sweet as sucrose. Your body breaks all sugars down to glucose in order to use it for energy.

Lactose and *galactose* are forms of sugar found in milk. You don't eat them in sugar form; they are part of all milk products.

Here's the simple rule: *Use sugar as sparingly as possible.* Follow this rule with other sweeteners, such as honey, brown sugar, maple syrup, corn syrup, or molasses, as well. They all react in your body the same way as sugar does.

A word about aspartame:

Aspartame, a popular artificial sweetener, is most often marketed as NutraSweet. The FDA approved it for use in 1974 and allowed its use in soft drinks in 1983. It replaced saccharine, another artificial sweetener, which studies suggested was carcinogenic in humans. It's 200 times sweeter than sugar and is now used in more than *7,000 food products.*

Although aspartame has been presumed safe for human use, Ralph G. Walton, M.D., from Western Reserve Care System, states that about a third of the population is vulnerable to an adverse reaction to aspartame. Of about a thousand nondrug-related cases of complaints about aspartame made to the FDA, 75 percent refer to problems with dizziness, headaches, numbness, vision changes, vomiting, muscle cramps and spasms, seizures, and abdominal pain.

Aspartame includes about 10 percent methanol (also called wood alcohol). This sweetener also contains formaldehyde and formic acid—known carcinogens, according to Dr. Julian Whitaker's *Health and Healing* newsletter (December 1994). You hasten your body's absorption of methanol if you use aspartame in hot drinks.

In view of all these facts, some health professionals have doubts about aspartame's safety. We recommend natural sweeteners such as honey or stevia. Although not well known in this country, stevia has been used by South American Indians for centuries. It is nontoxic, has medicinal value, and is sold in some health food stores.

SECRET 10: THEY HAVE CUT DOWN ON THEIR INTAKE OF SPICE AND SALT

Spice. Although there are many healthful herbs, few people seem to know that other seasonings, such as spices and condiments, can irritate the stomach and, in time, affect its lining, which then interferes with normal digestion.

Research done at Yale University and the Mexico Institute of Public Health has demonstrated a link between the use of chili peppers and gastric ulcers. Researchers asked those in the survey who lived in Mexico to report their use of chili peppers. When they compared nonusers with users, they discovered that those who ate chili peppers had 5.5 times greater risk of stomach cancer. Heavy users had 17 times greater risk of gastric cancer than nonusers.

Animal experiments done by Drs. Bernell and Marjorie Baldwin found that certain spices cause abnormal heart activity, increased blood pressure, and sometimes retching and vomiting. They cited mustard, cloves, cinnamon, and black pepper as causal agents in creating stomach lesions, although black pepper was four times as responsible as mustard.

Salt. The advice today from almost all nutritionists is, "Cut back or at least don't add any."

"But my food doesn't have any flavor otherwise," Richard Clark complains while liberally sprinkling on the salt.

"But you haven't even tasted it!" answers his wife.

"I've tasted it before," Richard says as he adds another generous amount.

What's wrong with that picture?

Salt isn't bad. In fact, we can't live without salt. But like Richard, you may be salting food out of habit and thus getting too much.

Let's look at salt and your body's needs.

Salt contains two minerals, sodium and chloride. Sodium (for which the word *salt* has become interchangeable) is the important one—it's in every cell in your body and in all your body fluids.

You probably don't need as much as you're using. Next to sugar, salt is our most overused and abused food additive. Most Americans eat 2 to 2 1/2 teaspoons every day. (That total includes hidden salt found in soups, canned vegetables, and other processed foods.) Your body can use only about 200 mg of salt a day—about 1/10 of a teaspoon. Even the Recommended Daily Allowance (RDA), which many health professionals consider exceedingly liberal concerning salt, suggests that adults not exceed 3,300 milligrams (about 1 3/5 teaspoons).

Consider this:

Higher sodium use interferes with your body's ability to remove fats from the bloodstream, which can contribute to cardiovascular diseases and possibly migraine headaches and stomach cancer.

How Salt Works against You

Although you need sodium, as soon as your intake becomes excessive, you open yourself up to problems. Salt stays in body tissues, which raises your blood pressure and causes you to retain water. Most people carry 5 to 7 extra pounds of water weight because of their overuse of salt. By decreasing your salt intake, you allow your body to shed that unneeded water.

Too much salt overworks your kidneys and can eventually cause serious problems. One reason for high salt use is that most Americans eat an abundance of meat and dairy products, which are naturally high in sodium. Our research shows that vegetarians generally eat a low-sodium, high-potassium diet, and they also tend to have considerably lower blood pressure than others their age.

Another health factor that is slowly gaining attention is the link between salt and stress. Overconsumption of salt produces more norepinephrine (a nervous system hormone), which makes people increasingly nervous and edgy.

About one-third of American adults have elevated blood pressure. For those over age sixty-five, the figure rises to 70 percent. By contrast, low blood pressure societies are those that have a low salt intake.

Did you know this?

Hypertension (high blood pressure)—aggravated by high salt intake—accounts for about half of the annual deaths in the United States.

"I can't stand tasteless food," is the common complaint. "I might as well be eating paper."

Does this sound like you? If so, you probably don't realize that your taste for salt isn't inborn. You learned to add salt. And the more salt you add to your food, the more you crave it. However, you can break the habit. Cut your salt intake back for three weeks and substitute healthful herbs. You'll be amazed how you can reeducate your taste buds.

Ronald Reagan successfully reeducated himself. When he was governor of California, his physician told him that he could live fifteen years longer if he stopped salting his food. And he changed his salt habit in less than a week, he said.

You can do it too!

As you cut back on what you add to food, also give yourself the benefit of avoiding certain processed foods. Stay away from or use little food that contains baking soda, baking powder, or MSG (monosodium glutamate). Also steer clear of salty snacks, anything pickled, presweetened cereals, and most canned vegetables.

Don't get discouraged. You can help yourself *cut down* on salt by:

- eating a variety of fresh, raw vegetables and fruit. (These foods also contain potassium, which helps lower blood pressure.)

- replacing salty snacks with celery sticks, carrot sticks, and sliced cucumbers.

- undercooking vegetables so they're crispy—and more satisfying.

- flavoring meals with natural flavor enhancers, such as parsley, lemon or lime juice, garlic, onions, tarragon, basil, curry, dill, fennel, ginger root, thyme, or turmeric.

- buying salt-free foods or at least foods low in salt. (Check your food labels for salt content. Almost all canned soups and vegetables are "salt mines.")

- cooking foods that are low in salt. Rice, for instance, needs little, if any, salt.

- removing the salt shaker from the table.

- filling your salt shaker with other flavorings.

- watching those sweet foods for hidden salt. (Yes, even products such as Jell-O chocolate pudding contain 1,200 mg of salt. One piece of cake gives you at least 1,000 mg.)

- avoiding or cutting back on such condiments as soy sauce, teriyaki sauce, Worcestershire sauce, catsup, mustard, and even bouillon cubes.

• ordering it your way when you eat out. Ask for food cooked as you want it cooked, not as they like to cook it. You are paying for it.

SECRET 11: MAYBE THEY TAKE VITAMIN AND MINERAL SUPPLEMENTS

Although supplements are still somewhat controversial, many nutritionists and health experts have found natural food supplements to be beneficial and are recommending their use. These experts point out how depleted much soil has become and how the food that is grown in it, then picked and packed early, may suffer a subsequent lack of nutrients. This topic goes beyond the scope of this book, but we recommend doing some research before you get heavily into supplements. Many of them are expensive; the wrong ones can throw off the balance of your system.

If you eat a wide variety of fruits, grain, vegetables, and nuts, you will probably get all the nutrients you need. If you choose to take vitamin supplements, think of them as a little extra life insurance— not as a substitute for healthy eating, but as an addition. Moderation, we believe, is important.

GETTING PRACTICAL

As you think about the generally unknown facts presented in this chapter, here are some ways you can incorporate them into your life.

1. Plan meals that don't use refined foods. You don't have to cut them all out at once, but make a plan so that you eventually eliminate such products as white bread, white macaroni, white rice, refined breakfast cereals, and instant potatoes.

2. Learn to plan your meals around complex carbohydrates. Use more whole-grain pasta, bread, cereals, and brown rice.

3. Get your sweets the natural way—from fresh and dried fruits.

4. Read labels. Avoid food products made up largely of refined ingredients.

5. Use milk substitutes—and there are many—made from rice or soy.

6. Try substitutes for butter and cheese or eat your bread plain.

7. When you eat out, visit the salad bar; there is usually a wide variety of fresh vegetables and fruits available, but avoid the vegetables seasoned with oil-based dressings, bacon bits, and croutons.

---

*I can expect to live longer and healthier
if I practice the secrets of good health.*

DRINK AS MUCH AS YOU WANT

"Do you drink enough water?"

. . .

Suppose you asked your friends that question. How do you think they'd respond?

"Of course I do," most would probably say.

Two problems, however, come with this question. The first is that the word *enough* is undefined. The second is in the meaning of the word *water*.

Before we explain, here is another question. Of all the essential elements your body requires, which does it need most—food or water? If you thought water, you answered correctly. Seventy percent of your weight is water. You could survive on your body's store of food for up to ten weeks; without water, you would live only a matter of days. Your health depends on many factors, but none is more important than water.

If you're average, you *don't* drink enough water. Most Americans drink only 3.3 glasses of water each day.

Your natural reaction may be to say, "Not so! I drink a lot of liquids."

True. If you're a typical American, you probably drink an abundance of fluids that include iced tea, colas, sweetened juices, and coffee. So you can say smugly, "No problem. I get plenty of fluid."

But drinking a lot of liquids isn't the same as drinking water. Many other liquids actually cause you to need *more* water. Their sugar and chemical additives force your body to work harder to separate those additives from the water.

Why Do We Need Water?

Most people don't give much consideration to water because it's so readily available. But drinking insufficient water can cause you to

- become irritable and even suffer minor depression
- have more body odor and bad breath
- produce a strong, unpleasant-smelling urine
- have difficulty keeping cool in hot weather because you don't have good insulation
- run the risk of kidney infections and kidney stones.

Lack of adequate water can slow down or harm your mental processes. In fact, without water, you couldn't even use the oxygen in the air because your lungs must be moist to do so. And you couldn't swallow, blink, or speak. You can't live when you lose as little as 20 percent of your body's water.

To get the idea of what it's like to function without enough water, imagine trying to take a bath in a cup of water.

Calculate Your Need for Water this Way:

Divide your weight by two. Think of that figure as the total number of ounces you need in a day. Divide that figure by eight to get the number of glasses you should drink. If you weigh 200 pounds, you need 100 ounces, or 12 1/2 glasses, of water daily.

For most people, the simplest advice is to drink eight 8-ounce glasses of just water each day. *Note:* If you're overweight, you need more water than those who have more slender bodies. For every extra twenty-five pounds you carry, you need to drink one extra glass of water.

Another method to measure the adequacy of your water intake is to monitor the color of your urine. Unless you have recently eaten something like asparagus or have taken a B vitamin capsule, the color of your urine should approximate the color of water from the tap. The darker your urine, the more water you need.

Thirst isn't a reliable guide to your body's needs. You usually need water long before your brain alerts you, so drink more than what you think you need to satisfy your thirst.

Every function of your body requires water.

The amount of water you drink directly relates to your ability to live healthfully and efficiently. You need this essential liquid both in your tissue cells and in the space surrounding the cells.

Healthy cell membranes maintain the distribution of water and allow the exchange of fluid and certain minerals through a mechanism scientists call osmotic pressure. If you are in good health, this osmotic pressure maintains about 60 percent of the water in your body inside your cells and the rest outside.

Every tissue, organ, and system operates in a liquid medium. Think of a car battery. It won't generate electricity to fire the engine if the water level gets too low. Your body depends on water even more than your car battery does. Dehydration causes your cells and tissues to malfunction.

Did you know that your body processes the equivalent of 2,500 gallons of water every day? (That's about 40,000 glasses!) Of course, most of it is recycled within your body. Your kidneys filter 400 gallons of blood daily.

And you lose a lot of water every day. The average person voids about five and a half glasses of fluid through urination and half a glass through the bowels.

As you exhale, you lose about two glasses' worth of moisture. Evaporation through the skin (perspiration) accounts for another two glasses. (If you're one of those individuals who perspire heavily, you lose more than two glasses.) Add those numbers together, and you'll see that you need at least ten glasses of water just to replace your normal loss every day. If you exercise, you need to replace even more.

How do you replace that lost water? The most obvious answer is to drink it—and drink plain water. You need *at least* five and a half 8-ounce glasses, but it would be better if you drank six to eight glasses. One way to remember how much you need is: "Drink five to stay alive; eight to feel great!" Most people get about three glasses of water through their food and up to another glass and a half as a by-product when their body burns or metabolizes food to provide energy. That's not very much, is it?

How Does Water Help Us?

- *Lubrication:* Saliva lubricates food; fluid bathes our eyes, lungs, and air passages.

- *Respiration:* Water in the nasal passages moistens air on its way to the lungs.

- *Circulation:* Water helps maintain blood consistency. Blood draws water from the cells around it. We need to replace that water in the cells.

- *Digestion:* Water helps enzymes in the stomach digest food.

- *Nourishment:* All nutrients reach cells in a fluid state.

- *Filtration:* Through the skin and kidneys, we excrete body poisons. The more water we drink, the less work our kidneys must do to eliminate body wastes. Water also helps prevent constipation.

- *Shock absorption:* Fluids in the joints cushion bones.

- *Temperature control:* We have two million sweat glands that continually moisten our skin. Evaporation from the skin helps cool the body to maintain an even temperature of 98.6°F. Water enables us to perspire freely.

We've already mentioned perspiration as one of the significant ways we steadily lose large amounts of water. Perspiration acts as a thermostat for controlling body temperature. The cooling effect of the evaporation of water from our skin allows us to maintain an even inner temperature regardless of environmental conditions. We tend to feel uncomfortable in humid weather because humidity inhibits this natural evaporation.

Thirst is the body's control mechanism for assuring an adequate water intake. Inadequate water replacement can result in water-depleted heat exhaustion. *Never ignore that possibility.*

You may be chronically dehydrated and not even know it. Cec Murphey knows this firsthand. For years he struggled with dry skin and resorted to creams and lotions to get rid of itching and scaling. One day, a friend casually remarked that the human body needs lubrication on the inside in order for the skin to get enough moisture.

"That's it," Cec said. He realized that he didn't drink much water, in part because he had once lived in an African nation where he had to filter and then boil water from the local river. "That spoiled the taste for me," he said.

He began forcing himself to drink more water. It took three months before he was drinking enough. His dry-skin problems have since disappeared.

DRINKING ENOUGH WATER

Rather than gulping down enough water once or twice a day, try to replace lost fluids frequently and in smaller amounts throughout the day. Water is something you seldom get too much of. You can even drink twice the amount you need and it won't hurt you. (Unless you have kidney or heart failure, your kidneys will get rid of any water you don't need.) However, it's not wise to flood your system. Your body functions best when there is a balance of the electrolyte system, and excessive water can upset this balance.

The Most Common Complaint about Drinking Adequate Water:

"But I'll have to keep running to the bathroom if I drink that much."

What's more important, the disadvantage of having to go to the bathroom a lot, or the advantage of your body's getting enough water? It's a small inconvenience for improved health.

Age, diet, activity level, and climate affect our water needs. Each of us is unique. Generally, infants, active people, and those living in warm-to-hot climates need more water than most adults who are sedentary or live in colder climates.

If we don't drink plenty of water before exercising, that deficiency eventually upsets our bodies' heat-control mechanism and forces our internal temperature to rise. When the body's temperature hits 102°F, severe exhaustion sets in. Drinking sufficient water can prevent this.

Here are two examples that show the importance of water replacement.

1. When ultra-marathon runner Stan Cottrell took a group of physicians on a one-day, 50-mile run, he insisted that everybody drink at least two glasses of water before they began. One doctor said, "I'm not thirsty."

   "Maybe not," Stan answered, "but by the time you are, it will be too late. You don't go on this run unless you drink first." Reluctantly, the physician complied.

   Stan led the physicians in the all-day run and included breaks and time for lunch along the way. The single factor he watched most closely, however, was that every doctor drank plenty of water. They completed their 50 miles. At the end, none of them felt either dehydrated or exhausted.

   Most people underestimate the amount of water they lose while doing activities. Some athletes lose up to five quarts during an exercise period or a game. If they don't replace it, not only do they feel severe fatigue, but they also deplete their bodies of salt. Eventually they may do severe damage to their bodies.

Sports advice:

- With adequate water intake, there is no need for sports drinks.

- Don't use salt pills except on the advice of a physician.

2. One major reason for the success of Sir Edmund Hillary's 1953 expedition in scaling Mount Everest was the forced drinking of water among his party. His men took along battery-operated ice melters and each member of the climbing team drank 5 to 7 pints of water a day.

By contrast, a Swiss party had tried the same climb only months earlier and had failed. Each person on that expedition had drunk less than 1 pint of water per day during the last three days of the unsuccessful climb.

> **Think about water this way:**
> The world's surface consists of about 70 percent water, which is about the same amount as the human body. If you want to be healthy, keep your water level up to 70 percent.

WHEN TO DRINK

It's best to drink water up to 30 minutes before a meal. Wait an hour after a meal before drinking again. The only time *not* to drink water is during a meal. Water dilutes the digestive juices in the mouth, makes the food mix in the stomach too thin, and impairs digestion. Stomach enzymes work best in a concentrated, undiluted mixture.

Another reason to avoid drinking during a meal is that people who take a lot of water with their meals tend to chew less. They wash food down instead of chewing it, and bolting down food is a causative factor in overeating.

If you miss drinking water with meals, try adding foods like watermelon. The higher the liquid content of your food, the less you'll feel the need to drink.

Very cold or extremely hot beverages, when taken with meals, have a tendency to arrest the digestive process until the stomach can raise or lower the temperature of its contents to body temperature. Avoid ice-cold water. It decreases the surface blood in the stomach and requires too much energy to warm it up to the temperature necessary for digestion.

WATER AND WEIGHT CONTROL

If you're concerned about your weight, remember that water contains no calories. If you drink eight glasses of water every day, it can help you avoid gaining excess pounds. Doing so may even help you lose some weight.

Hungry or thirsty?

Many who struggle with their weight think they're hungry when they're actually thirsty. The next time you feel strong hunger cravings between meals, drink one full glass of water. If your hunger lessens within minutes, you were simply thirsty.

Water is one of the best diuretics—and certainly the most healthful. If you feel waterlogged (not because of heart failure), drink more water. Some people mistakenly believe they will retain less water if they drink less. What they don't realize is that a sodium imbalance causes water retention. However, if they drink additional water, they will flush some of the excess salt from their systems. So drinking more water actually helps to avoid that bloated feeling.

Water and Health Control

Most people overlook water's power to aid their bodies in overcoming viral and bacterial infections. For example:

- Drinking hot water can function as a natural decongestant for upper respiratory infections. When battling a cold, drink your water warm and benefit from God's natural decongestant.

- When fighting a cold or flu, or even a headache, drink a glass of water every ten minutes for an hour. The theory here is that a hydrated body is best able to assist the immune system to help itself. Note: This recommendation is for one hour, not longer. Even when drinking water, moderation is an important health principle. Don't throw your body chemistry out of balance by drinking too much.

GETTING PRACTICAL

How do you get enough water? Drinking enough water is a habit you have to learn. Here are ten things to help you develop that habit.

1. If you have not been drinking eight glasses of water every day, increase the amount you drink *gradually*. Allow yourself at least two weeks to reach that goal.

2. Drink one or two glasses of water the first thing every morning. While you slept, your body continued to function. Even though your body's need for water diminished somewhat during sleep, you have lost water in at least three ways: through the kidneys, through the pores of the skin, and through exhaled air. After eight hours of such activity, a low level of dehydration has set in. Start the day by replenishing what you lost during the night.

3. Drink at least one glass of water between breakfast and lunch. Drink at least another glass in the middle of the afternoon. Drink a final glass in the evening.

4. Keep a two-quart jar or container of water at your desk or workplace. Sip from it throughout the day.

5. If you don't drink water because it doesn't taste good to you, add a little lemon, orange, or mint to flavor it.

6. If you have a drinking fountain nearby, fill your glass several times a day and drink it all. Take a drink every time you pass a water fountain. Eleven or twelve good gulps equal 8 ounces of water.

7. When you take part in an exercise program, remind yourself to drink a glass of water before and after. (Some people also carry water with them during their exercise.)

8. Instead of coffee breaks, give yourself water breaks.

9. Avoid drinking water with your meals. Instead, drink up to 30 minutes before and begin again one hour after meals.

10. Don't count alcohol, colas, coffee, and other drinks for your total water intake. Forty-five percent of Americans drink coffee as their primary liquid intake, and 78 percent have turned to soft drinks. This figure exceeds 100 percent because some people drink both. If you think drinking alcohol will contribute to your water intake, you might be surprised to learn that you need eight ounces of water to metabolize one ounce of pure alcohol.

Because I want to live healthier and longer,
I will drink at least eight glasses of water each day.

JUST ANOTHER DRINK?

CHAPTER 6

QUESTION: WHAT are America's most common addictive drinks?

. . .

Answer: Caffeinated drinks, such as soft drinks and coffee (while alcohol is the major drug problem, far more people drink coffee or caffeinated drinks).

About 80 percent of the adult population of the United States drink some kind of beverage that contains caffeine. If you're a typical American, you probably use up to 300 mg of caffeine every day, which you can achieve with only three cups of coffee. At least 20 percent of Americans use more than 350 mg daily—a level that constitutes physical dependency. Together, Americans drink the equivalent of 400 million cups of coffee *every* day.

How Much Caffeine?

- The average cup of instant coffee contains about 65 mg (percolated coffee has about 110).
- Tea and most soft drinks contain 30 to 65 mg a serving.
- Hot chocolate beverages provide about 5 mg of caffeine.
- Chocolate candy holds between 10 and 40 mg per 2-ounce bar.

Someone once said, "Cars run on gas, lights on electricity, and Americans on coffee." Despite declines in the amount of coffee Americans consume—much of the under-thirty crowd is turning to colas—we still drink more than half of the coffee produced in the world. By contrast, 74 percent of those in the Live-Longer Lifestyle studies maintain a caffeine-free diet.

Children and caffeine:

Based on body weight, children up to five years of age are the heaviest consumers of caffeine. Young children who drink one can of caffeinated soda receive the caffeine equivalent of four cups of coffee in an adult. For a seven-year-old child, three cans of regular Coke are equivalent to eight cups of coffee to an adult.

WHY DO PEOPLE DRINK CAFFEINE?

Most people drink caffeinated beverages for three reasons.

First, the effects of caffeine are experienced quickly. The body readily absorbs it. Caffeine reaches its peak level in the blood within thirty minutes.

Second, it's available almost everywhere. Can you think of any function where the coffeepot isn't present? Business meetings, clubs, associations—somebody always provides the coffee. Church socials probably wouldn't function without the brew. Many churches now have a coffee hour either before or after their morning worship hour. And have you ever attended an all-day seminar that didn't involve at least one coffee break?

Third, they like the feel and taste of hot liquids.

EFFECTS OF CAFFEINE

1. *There are no positive effects of caffeine.* Temporarily, you get an extra charge of energy. However, it's "borrowed" energy. You get it

now, but later you have to pay it back by living with a lower energy level. You can take more caffeine to put off the "payback," but eventually, like all big debts, you have to pay for it.

When you ingest caffeine, it doubles the level of adrenaline in your bloodstream. That's why it shocks your system. The adrenaline causes your liver to rapidly dump glucose (blood sugar) into your bloodstream.

Caffeine activates your body's self-preservation faculties. The energy you get is the kind intended to protect you from danger in emergencies. This stresses your whole body, especially your nervous system. Adrenaline produces a high level of tension that you can normally relieve only by physical action. If you don't take physical action, this tension can last for hours and produce headache, nervousness, sleeplessness, and other unpleasant symptoms of stress.

2. *Caffeine harms your body.* It unbalances your autonomic nervous system, which controls the function of every major organ in your body. It also

- elevates blood sugar (gives the feeling of an energy surge)

- aggravates hypoglycemia

- increases blood pressure

- stimulates the central nervous system and can cause you to overcome your body's need for rest

- can cause irregular heart beat

- increases urinary calcium and magnesium losses, which can decrease bone health

- constricts blood vessels

- increases stomach acid secretion, which can aggravate a stomach ulcer

- can cause tremors, irritability, and nervousness

- disrupts sleep and causes insomnia

- increases anxiety and depression

- heightens symptoms of premenstrual syndrome (PMS)

3. *Heavy caffeine consumption elevates your serum cholesterol and increases your risk of heart disease.*

Did you know this?

If you're an average caffeine user and you stop your caffeine intake, it will probably mean about a 10 percent decrease in your cholesterol level.

Although animal studies have linked heavy coffee use with colon, bladder, and ovarian cancer, it has not been until recently that human studies have been conducted. One was a twenty-year study at Loma Linda University (1960–1980) involving 23,912 people, and the results definitely linked coffee consumption to colon, bladder, and bowel cancer. Even two daily cups of coffee increase the risk of fatal colon cancer or fatal bladder cancer.

4. *Caffeinism syndrome—a condition indistinguishable from anxiety neurosis—can result when people ingest large doses of caffeine (650–1,000 mg a day).* Those who are caffeine-sensitive report anxiety and severe depression after only 300 mg. Children allowed high doses of caffeine display hyperactive behavior.

The principal of a Christian boarding academy made an interesting observation. One of the rules he inherited from the previous administration was "no caffeine-containing soda on bus trips." On the first trip he supervised, he enforced the rule en route to their destination, even though the teenagers grumbled and complained. The students were orderly and polite.

On the way home, when the kids were dead tired, he announced he would not enforce the "no caffeine soda rule," and at the next stop almost all the students got back on the bus with Coke, Pepsi, Dr. Pepper, or Mountain Dew. Almost immediately, bedlam broke out. The teens' disruptive loud voices and hyperactive behavior made it impossible for others to sleep or for the faculty to control them. It only took one experiment for the principal to realize the wisdom of the rule about no caffeinated drinks.

5. *Caffeine tends to make you more talkative* by increasing your flow of thoughts. Caffeine also causes some people to become more impulsive and to have difficulty listening.

6. *Caffeine has no effect on the fatigue mechanisms of the body.* The relief from fatigue people experience after taking caffeine is merely a *perception.* They have the illusion they are rested and use their energy reserves to live out this illusion. When the effects of caffeine wear off, most people are far more tired than before. Sometimes mild depression follows.

Here are two of many research experiments that show the effects of caffeine.

1. *Typists.* Researchers tested a group of typists who had used no caffeine for at least two weeks. Their typing was accurate, and they correctly estimated their speed.

   In the second part of the test, each participant drank two cups of coffee. The typists' accuracy decreased considerably. However, *in their self-evaluations, they thought they were doing much better in speed and accuracy* than when they had not used caffeine. The apparent improvement they felt in performance after imbibing caffeine was illusionary. This led researchers to say that although caffeine stimulates you when you are rested, it doesn't improve your performance beyond what you could accomplish with adequate rest and no caffeine.

2. *Spiders.* Dr. Mervyn G. Hardinge, formerly dean of the School of Public Health, Loma Linda University, injected spiders with caffeine to see how it would affect their behavior in spinning their webs. He gave them a dose equivalent to two cups of coffee for a 155-pound man. They wove webs of strange, non-symmetrical patterns.

HIDDEN CAFFEINE

You may think you are bypassing this caffeine-dependent lifestyle because you don't drink coffee or colas. But caffeine lurks in many products today. Check the label; you'll find caffeine even in such drinks as Mountain Dew and Dr. Pepper. You'll also find it added to diet drinks, such as Tab.

Caffeine and Medicine

Are you aware that Excedrin and several other analgesics contain as much caffeine as two cups of coffee? The aspirin relieves your pain, and the caffeine gives you an upbeat feeling.

Read the labels on cold medicines and amaze yourself as you see caffeine as a major ingredient.

"But what if I switch to decaf coffee?" people like Richard Clark often ask. "Won't that take care of the problems?"

Maybe. Some decaffeination is done naturally, through the sun or water, and it probably has no harmful effects. But another method is a chemical-leeching process, which could be harmful.

"It's the comfort of hot liquid people really want," says Dr. John Reinhold. "So why not switch to one of three dozen varieties of herbal tea? That way, you get the comfort and you know it's safe."

Some people have stopped drinking Coke or Pepsi, switched to Sprite or other "un-colas," and believe they've eliminated the problems. True, they don't get the caffeine, but they're still drinking harmful chemicals. For instance, high levels of phosphorus contribute to problems such as osteoporosis and poor teeth. We think it's wiser to avoid all soft drinks.

Getting Practical

Here are easy tips to help you reduce caffeine in your diet or eliminate it altogether.

1. Drink water, herbal tea, or juices made from fruits and vegetables.

2. If you use chocolate products, use them sparingly. Carob is a decent alternative.

3. If you want a soft drink, why not make your own? Mix club soda or sparkling mineral water with freshly squeezed fruit juice. When you do this, you'll notice your drink is not as sweet as the commercial products. Resist the temptation to add sugar.

4. Try coffee substitutes, such as Postum, which have been available in grocery stores for most of this century. Other substitutes are readily available in health food stores. They don't taste like coffee, but they do make excellent hot replacements. Or you might try:

    • Bambu (made from chicory, figs, wheat, malted barley, and acorns)

    • Kaffree Roma (roasted malt barley, barley, and chicory)

    • Pionier (barley, figs, and chicory)

    • Sipp (roasted barley, chicory, rye, chickpea and fig)

KICKING THE HABIT

If you're addicted to caffeine, expect some withdrawal symptoms when you quit. The first symptoms usually begin 12 to 24 hours after your last caffeine intake. Symptoms vary with individuals, but may include headache, fatigue, apathy, and possibly anxiety. These symptoms usually peak at 36 hours. Normally, it takes about a week for full recovery.

People use different methods to quit. Some stop "cold turkey"; others succeed by gradually reducing the amount of their intake.

The most successful way to win over caffeine is to stop immediately. It's not easy for most people, but they will recover faster from withdrawal symptoms this way. If you choose to go cold turkey, sudden caffeine withdrawal may feel awful but presents no health problems.

If you choose gradual withdrawal, set a timetable for yourself. For example, if you drink lots of coffee, decide to drink only one cup in the morning and one in the afternoon. During the next week, leave a quarter of the coffee in your cup. The following week, drink only half a cup in the morning and half a cup in the afternoon. Then cut down to a quarter cup each time. The following week, eliminate the afternoon quarter cup. By then you can probably drop the habit totally. You can use this same process with other sources of caffeine. Unfortunately, this method is not usually as successful as stopping suddenly. It may also prolong the withdrawal symptoms for weeks.

If you decide to kick the caffeine habit, water can be a good ally. Caffeine overly stimulates the kidneys and causes an excess excretion of water. However, if you drink large amounts of water, you can help to flush the caffeine residues from your system and reduce the period of withdrawal symptoms.

As an adult, if you drink caffeine in any form, it generally takes 5 to 7 hours to eliminate it from your body (or up to 20 hours if you're pregnant; newborns need several days). The time required depends on a number of variables, such as your age, sex, hormone levels, medications, and whether you smoke.

MINIMIZING WITHDRAWAL EFFECTS

Eat no solid food, soup, or milk for the first 24 hours. Drink only fruit juice and water. Be sure you drink a total of at least eight to ten glasses of liquid. This will flush the caffeine from your body. Drink throughout the day because the energy you receive from each glass of juice only lasts about two hours.

Juice helps you combat fatigue, the most common withdrawal symptom. Fruit juices also contain the vitamins and minerals you need to help your system recover from the effects of caffeine. However, if you are diabetic or have heart trouble or any other chronic condition, consult your physician before drinking large quantities of juice—or even water.

If you have headaches (which isn't unusual), use a noncaffeinated analgesic, such as Tylenol or Advil. You can expect headaches to disappear in 24 to 36 hours. Fatigue and irritability can last three or four days before your normal energy level returns.

You may experience dizziness, sleepiness during the day, and perhaps even mild depression. These symptoms usually disappear within 24 hours.

Remember that eliminating caffeine from your diet is worth the effort. You will feel better. You will be taking control of your life. You will be taking one more step toward a longer and healthier life.

---

*Because I choose to live a healthier,
longer life, I don't depend on stimulants.*

THAT OTHER DRINK

CHAPTER 7

"HEY, ONE glass of alcohol or so a day is supposed to be good for you. Right?"

· · ·

I'm sure you've heard that argument. But is it true?

Before we give you the answer, let's look carefully at alcohol and its usage. And by alcohol we mean all forms—from beer to wine to the "hard" alcoholic drinks, such as whiskey or vodka.

Less than 5 percent of those in the Live-Longer Lifestyle study group drink alcohol. By contrast, surveys indicate that 10 million Americans consider themselves social drinkers, with another 10 million classified as alcoholics. Since the early 1980s, alcohol consumption in the United States has declined. Even so, alcohol presents the greatest drug problem in the world.

Although American consumption has declined, one age group—those under twenty-five—has actually increased its alcohol intake.

Before you take another drink, consider this: Alcohol is responsible for 45 billion dollars' worth of industrial losses a year, from sickness to poor decision making. Alcohol is involved in 50 percent of all traffic fatalities and 30 percent of aircraft accidents. Plus it's linked to 66 percent of all violent crimes. You're probably aware of the alarming figures about the effects of alcohol. Some speak of alcohol as the most dangerous *legal* drug in the world.

If you're concerned about healthy living, here is the first fact you need to know: Alcohol does nothing for your body except make you feel relaxed and uninhibited. True, some researchers have reported the value of alcohol in limited amounts. They claim that it raises levels of HDL, the good cholesterol that protects against artery disease. However, alcohol also raises levels of HDL3, a subgroup that doesn't offer this protection. But why take a chance when at the same time alcohol can cause irreversible liver damage?

Like caffeine and nicotine, alcohol *is* a drug. That means it has the potential to be addictive. Beyond the addictive element, what about the health hazards associated with it?

In the examples below, you will read of the effects of what we call "excessive amounts." Yet you'll also see that even imbibing small amounts can begin the physical damage. So think seriously about the effects of alcohol on health.

1. *Alcohol reduces the heart's working capacity.* The late Nathan Pritikin said that just two cocktails cut a normal heart's activity by 20 percent for about 24 hours. Those who are two-drink-a-day persons have already deprived themselves of 1/5 of their hearts.

2. *Alcohol raises blood pressure, which can lead to strokes.* In one study, drinkers had twice the rate of strokes of nondrinkers, and heavy drinkers experienced five times more strokes.

3. *Alcohol interferes with the absorption of calcium from food.* Social drinkers are two-and-a-half times more likely to develop osteoporosis than nondrinkers.

4. *Alcohol has been linked to the development of a variety of cancers—* including cancer of the throat, mouth, larynx, pharynx, esophagus, bladder, breast, pancreas, head, neck, and liver. Urethane is a cancer-causing agent that forms in alcoholic drinks as the result of naturally occurring chemical reactions.

5. *Alcoholic beverages have been found to contain pesticide residues from sprayed fruits or grains.* Some people develop allergic reactions, and many drinkers are amazed when they learn they are allergic to ingredients in beer, wine, and distilled spirits. These allergies can affect their skin or gastrointestinal and respiratory systems.

6. *Alcohol is high in calories.* This is what gives some the appropriately named "beer belly." Alcohol is an empty-calorie beverage that contains no vitamins.

7. *Alcohol contributes to the loss of white blood cells.* It weakens your immune system's ability to fight off infections and cancerous cells.

8. *Alcohol interferes with the work of your liver.* A healthy liver can handle only two or three teaspoons of alcohol an hour and may take as long as 24 hours to eliminate the alcohol and its by-products from just one drink.

9. *Excessive alcohol usage can lead to cirrhosis of the liver*—the seventh leading cause of death in the United States. Cirrhosis is a scarring of the liver where normal cells are damaged and unable to carry on their vital functions. It's an irreversible condition.

10. *Alcohol has a definite link to birth defects.* In the early 1980s the Surgeon General reported that FAS (fetal alcohol syndrome) causes permanent physical and mental damage to the fetus. Not only pregnant mothers have been implicated. A father who is drunk at his child's conception also runs the risk of producing a child with FAS. (Even low levels of alcohol can have negative neurological effects on the unborn.)

11. *Alcohol is now being associated with several cancers.* Because of alcohol's irritating effects on body tissues, a strong relationship is developing between alcohol use and cancer of the mouth, tongue, throat, esophagus, stomach, liver, lung, pancreas, colon (large intestine), and rectum.

Despite all the evidence, recent research suggests that "moderate" use of wine reduces the risk of heart attacks. This information has received wide dissemination. But how reliable are those results?

Did you know that health officials have *not* endorsed the consumption of one or two daily alcoholic drinks? In 1992 the U.S. Bureau of Alcohol, Tobacco, and Firearms forced the removal of E. and J. Gallo's claim from their burgundy that it was a suitable companion for a healthy meal. The bureau said that the promotional representations on reduced heart disease were a "misleading curative and therapeutic claim" and were inconsistent with the required warning labels on wine.

Before you pick up your glass, Richard, you might also consider that, because of heavier alcohol consumption, French men are three times more likely than American men to die of cancer of the esophagus.

And, Carol, both French men and women are more than twice as likely to die of stomach cancer—the types linked to alcohol consumption. The French also die of cirrhosis and chronic liver disease at almost twice the rate of Americans.

Why not grape juice?

Dr. Leron Creasy of Cornell University has identified a chemical in wine called resveratrol that may help to reduce heart disease. He then sampled Welch's grape juice and discovered that it contained *more* resveratrol than 60 percent of the wines he originally sampled.

GETTING PRACTICAL

1. Give your body alcohol-free days. If you tend to have a drink every day, cut back by going without alcohol two or three days a week.

2. Learn healthier ways to relax. Many say they have a social drink to unwind from the emotional stress of life. Ironically, excessive

drinking reduces the body's ability to absorb certain B vitamins that help the nervous system deal effectively with stress. Exercise is the best way to relax because it releases morphine-like chemicals in your brain called endorphins. These endorphins give you a sense of well-being, and they also strengthen your entire physical system.

3. Avoid situations or circumstances that would make you succumb to drinking. For example, if you drink when you are depressed, find other ways to cope with your depression, such as a regular exercise program.

4. Switch to one of the many nonalcoholic "taste-alikes" that are growing increasingly popular as substitutes for beer, wine, or cocktails.

5. Get help if you have trouble cutting down. If you can't cut down, or find yourself saying, "Next week I'll be in a better position to cut back," you may need professional help. Denial is the common symptom of *habitual* alcohol use.

I choose to live healthier and longer,
and I avoid the things that hinder that goal.

JUST DO IT!

CHAPTER 8

WOULD YOU be willing to take a pill if it could guarantee

- a 50 percent decrease in the risk of heart disease?

- lower blood pressure and cholesterol levels?

- some protection against cancer, diabetes, and osteoporosis?

- dramatically improved oxygen delivery to muscle cells?

- decreased mental anxiety and depression?

- increased energy?

- a longer life with improved quality of life?

Of course! And you would probably be willing to pay a significant sum for it.

That "pill" is called exercise.

Despite all the publicity about the effects of exercise, estimates are that only one out of five individuals "take the pill" on a regular basis. Some suggest that the rate could be even lower.

Exercise isn't a cure-all. But it is one of the essential components to treating our bodies as God's temple. A regular exercise program is an indispensable major part of living a decade longer and healthier.

Moderate exercise is the answer. In fact, while moderate exercise tends to strengthen the function of the immune system, too much exercise lowers it. When you begin an exercise program, work smart. Gradually increase the length and strenuousness of your exercise rather than overtaxing your unconditioned body. If you have any questions about your physical fitness or the possible negative consequences of exercising because of your health status, get your doctor's approval first.

All movement, regardless of how little, is beneficial. Moderate exercise will keep your body in good physical condition; vigorous exercise will strengthen your heart muscle and add months or years to your life; whereas excessive exercise that overtaxes your body is detrimental to both health and longevity.

We advocate walking 2 or 3 miles, or for 30 or 45 minutes, four or five times a week. This is probably the best exercise that most people can participate in without injury. It's also something they can participate in for most of their lives. Walkers comment that they not only get the exercise they need, but they can also study the trees, marvel at nature, listen to the birds, and even converse with friends. Walking to most people is less boring than pedaling the stationary bicycle.

Exercise in the open air offers higher benefits than indoor exercises because of your exposure to the benefits of sunlight and negative ions in the air.

Ask yourself:

Would it be worthwhile to spend 30 minutes a day for five days a week (about 5,200 hours during 40 years of adult life) exercising in order to live 80,000 hours—10 healthy years—longer?

The point of fitness is to be good to yourself. Do the things for your body that make you feel better and enable you to live a healthier life.

BENEFITS OF EXERCISE

Here are a number of reasons to start a regular exercise program.

1. *Exercise improves the cardiovascular system of the body.* People who are physically active tend to weigh less and have lower blood pressure and lower serum cholesterol levels. This makes for a lower risk for heart disease.

2. *Exercise prevents disease.* An ancient proverb says, "Every man has two doctors, his right leg and his left." An exercise program, in addition to fighting diseases of the heart and blood vessels, strengthens the body against such deadly diseases as cancer, diabetes, and osteoporosis.

   Exercise and cancer. Exercise guards against cancer because it helps to keep the immune system strong—which is the body's primary defense against cancer cells. Because exercise speeds up metabolism and the elimination of wastes, it helps prevent colon and rectal cancers.

   Exercise and diabetes. Those who exercise vigorously can reduce their risk of diabetes by 42 percent. Overweight people benefit the most, even if they don't lose weight. Vigorous activity appears to work equally well for men and women in heading off adult-onset diabetes, which accounts for 95 percent of the four-teen million cases of diabetes in America.

   Exercise and osteoporosis. Bones can't be strengthened without regular, weight-bearing exercise, such as walking. To retain their minerals, bones need to be pressed, pushed, pulled, and twisted against gravity.

3. *Exercise improves self-image, tones muscles, and helps maintain an ideal weight.* Exercise gives a sense of personal accomplishment. This spills over into other areas of life, including the increase of self-esteem. All effective weight-loss programs involve some form of an exercise program.

4. *Exercise relieves stress without drugs.* A natural mood elevator, exercise stimulates the pituitary gland at the base of the brain to release hormones called endorphins into the bloodstream. These have a tranquilizing effect on the body and are released after about 30 minutes of aerobic exercise. They elevate mood and increase the body's threshold for pain. That's why exercise relaxes tense muscles and releases pent-up negative emotions—reducing anger and frustration.

5. *Exercise charges the brain and nerve cells with electric energy.* It gives better balance between the voluntary and autonomic nervous systems.

6. *Exercise benefits every part of the body* because it

   - aids digestion and promotes intestinal activity, reducing gas and constipation

   - strengthens muscles, bones, and ligaments

   - prevents the loss of bone minerals and thus prevents osteoporosis

   - brings a physiological balance to the endocrine system, helping the pituitary, pancreas, adrenals, and sex glands to function more efficiently

   - sharpens mental powers and increases the capacity to think

   - beautifies the figure and complexion

   - produces more energy than the exercise uses

   - increases endurance and delays the onset of fatigue

7. *Exercise benefits longevity.* The results of an unpublished study on longevity that Jan presented in 1988 at the American Public Health convention concluded that those who exercised regularly outlived those who didn't exercise—by five years.

WALKING IS BEST

Brisk walking is the best, easiest, and cheapest activity you can do. If you feel sluggish or have been under stress, a long walk can relieve the tension and take you toward an attitude of serenity. Walk erect in the open air at a comfortable pace. Walking is easier on the joints than running, and there is less likelihood of injury. Do a brief warmup of stretching exercises before you start to walk. Start slowly and decide on an easily reached distance. Over the days ahead, gradually increase your speed and distance.

MAKE EXERCISE FUN

When Jan worked at Loma Linda University, he usually swam during his lunch hour. When he returned to work for the afternoon, his body felt refreshed, alert, and energetic, as if he were starting his day again in the morning. That feeling continued for the rest of the day.

At Loma Linda University, a group of fifty medical students volunteered for a ten-day experimental program. All of them ate a diet high in cholesterol, fat, protein, and carbohydrates. Then they chose an exercise program, such as volleyball, tennis, swimming, or running. Their daily blood cholesterol levels were taken. Within three days, the cholesterol level of every student had dropped. By the end of the first week, the drop was substantial.

Then the volunteers stopped their activities. Within days, the cholesterol in their blood returned to the pre-experiment levels. In some cases, the levels were a little higher.

For the next phase of the experiment, the students worked out on treadmills. Now they had exercise, but not in an enjoyable form. They exercised as strenuously as they had in their chosen sports. Again, each day their blood cholesterol levels were taken. Then came the surprise. Their cholesterol failed to drop. In most cases, levels went *up.* However, once they returned to physical activities they enjoyed, the students saw a drop in cholesterol *in every case.* This experiment shows the importance of attitude. A negative attitude produced enough stress to counteract the benefits of exercise.

This brings you to a choice: Either learn to like your form of exercise, or change your activity to one that you do like.

SIMPLE, EASY-TO-DO EXERCISES

Exercise can become a regular part of your lifestyle if you open yourself to the possibilities around you. Here are a few of what we call bonus exercises.

1. When you go to the mall, park as far from the stores as you can. The extra few minutes to and from your vehicle could amount to half a mile of walking.

2. Use the stairs. At work or other offices, use the stairway whenever possible. This provides an excellent cardiovascular exercise. If you have stairs in your home or apartment, find excuses to go up and down them several times a day.

3. If you have a cordless phone, pace while you talk.

4. Hide the TV remote control.

5. If you use a shopping cart at the grocery store, push it to the end of the aisle and leave it. Walk up and down the aisle, pick up the items you want, and take them to your cart. After you have checked out, push the cart to your car. Then walk all the way back to the store with the empty cart. It's not far, but it means more body movement.

6. Enlist a friend and walk together at least two miles a day.

7. Do stretching exercises in the open air.

Muscles were made for movement. Without exercise, you begin to deteriorate slowly. As with an undriven car, rest brings rust. And this physical decline can also bring mental and emotional decline.

MOTIVATING YOURSELF TO EXERCISE

Choosing the right exercise is as important as actually exercising. The Live-Longer Lifestyle studies have shown that people must enjoy the activity they get involved in to gain full benefit from it. Exercise can be a pleasurable, even exhilarating, activity.

1. Think of exercise as an act of spirituality. (It is.) At one time, many Christians took a strong interest in fitness. They considered that taking care of their bodies was preparation for the second coming of Jesus Christ. They seriously memorized verses that called human bodies the temples of God. One verse even says that those who destroy the temple will themselves be destroyed. (See 1 Cor. 3:17.) Consequently, to them, the care of the body was as significant as prayer or any other spiritual activity.

2. Challenge yourself to exercise. Set a goal. Say, "Today I will walk for five minutes. A brief walk will refresh me and make me feel better." After a few days, increase your time to 10 minutes. Continue lengthening your exercise time by 5 minutes until you walk 30 minutes a day. Do this four or five times a week, and try to keep it up on a regular basis. Continue increasing your time and distance until your final objective is reached.

3. Begin slowly and gradually. Don't push too hard or too fast in the beginning. If you do, you'll tend to burn out quickly and give up.

4. Get into a regular program. Exercise at a set time each day.

5. Stay with your exercise. If you choose walking, and the weather is bad, walk inside a mall or the airport terminal.

6. Exercise because you love life. As you begin to reap the benefits of fitness, you will spontaneously learn to love your exercise program—if you choose the right one.

Because I want to live longer and healthier,
I make exercise a high priority.

A STOP IN TIME

FIVE DAYS ago, three jumbo jets crashed in California. More than a thousand people died in the separate crashes. Four days ago, three more planes crashed outside Miami. Everyone on board each plane died. Three days ago, a plane crashed in Denver, another in Boston, and one in Atlanta. In each crash, everyone on board died. Yesterday another thousand people died in airline tragedies. So far today, two planes have crashed. In the past five days alone, the average daily death count has been one thousand people.

. . .

These air crashes didn't happen, but suppose they had. Suppose that *every day of this year,* an average of one thousand people died in plane-related accidents. What would the fallout of those deaths be?

A cry of panic from the public, certainly. Demands for investigation. The warning would spread across the nation, "Don't fly!" Fewer people would buy tickets for air travel. Congress would intervene with investigations and pass emergency regulations for the airline industry. From every section of the population would rise a clamor to put an end to such tragic deaths.

Yet tragedy strikes just as viciously every single day in the United States. At least one thousand people die *every day* from a preventable, self-inflicted cause. A few people have raised the alarm, but most people have no idea how serious this problem is. They hear reports but have yet to absorb the seriousness of what they hear or read.

C. Everett Koop, former U.S. Surgeon General, used the analogy of daily plane crashes to make the point that smoking continues to be the leading cause of disease, disability, and premature death in this country.

Here are a few facts about smoking:

- Male smokers are three times more likely than nonsmokers to die of lung cancer between the ages of forty-four and seventy.

- Of the women under age fifty who suffer heart attacks, 84 percent are smokers.

- Every day more than three thousand American teenagers smoke for the first time. If they continue—and most do—they expose themselves to the risk of lung cancer, heart disease, strokes, and other tobacco-related illnesses.

- Cigarettes kill more Americans annually than AIDS, cocaine, heroin, alcohol, automobiles, homicide, suicide, and fire combined.

- Thirty percent of all cancer deaths (including 90 percent of those with lung cancer) result from smoking.

- Smoking more than twenty cigarettes a day doubles the likelihood of developing cataracts.

- Medicare will spend one trillion dollars over the next twenty years treating people hospitalized for diseases caused by the abuse of tobacco, alcohol, and drugs.

- More than 36 percent of Medicare recipients are former smokers, and nearly 20 percent smoke now.

BENEFITS OF QUITTING

"Smoking cessation represents the single most important step that smokers can take to enhance the length and quality of their lives."—C. Everett Koop[1]

Hear the good news: Unless there is already onset of disease, it doesn't matter how long you have smoked, you can enjoy good health after quitting. The data from the Live-Longer life table analysis indicates that if smokers quit before they reach the age of fifty, their life expectancy goes up an average of an additional 1.5 years. By the time they reach seventy, there is virtually no difference in longevity between them and those who have never smoked.

After fifteen years of nonsmoking, your risk of death falls to nearly the same level as those who have never smoked—unless irreversible damage occurred before you stopped, such as lung disease or cancer.

REASONS TO QUIT SMOKING

1. You'll have fewer days of illness, fewer health complaints, better overall health status, and fewer lung problems.

2. You'll spend less money for cold remedies, health care, and life insurance.

3. Your chances of a stroke decline quickly after you quit.

4. If you quit smoking at age fifty, you have half the risk of dying in the next fifteen years of those who continue to smoke.

5. You're 50 percent less likely to suffer from impotence than are smokers.

6. Smoking cessation decreases the risk of lung and other cancers, heart attack, stroke, and chronic lung disease.

Good News for Smokers

If you're one of those smokers who has tried everything and you still can't quit, here's a medical breakthrough!

Dr. Linda Hyder Ferry of Loma Linda University has discovered a safe prescription medication called bupropion—a mild stimulant antidepressant that mimics the effects of nicotine on the brain. It is the first FDA-approved, nonaddicting medication for smoking cessation. Bupropion (brand name: Zyban) decreases cravings in people who still smoke. After they quit, it decreases their nicotine-withdrawal symptoms.

GETTING PRACTICAL

1. Plan to win—but plan it your way. Studies show that 90 percent of smokers quit on their own. Others do better by enrolling in clinics or joining support groups.

2. One lost battle isn't ultimate defeat. Don't plan to fail, but if you give in and smoke a cigarette, don't get discouraged. This is when so many say, "So much for good intentions," and return to smoking at their previous level. Instead, remind yourself that you can quit again and win the next battle. Each victory will take you a little closer to ultimate triumph over your addiction.

3. Concentrate on the benefits of victory. You are taking charge of your life. The minute you stop smoking, you begin to regenerate your body and repair the damage done to your heart, lungs, and body tissues.

4. Make a list of reasons you want to quit. Read your list at least once a day. For instance, you may write the following:

   • I want to have a healthy body.
   • I want to be able to walk two miles a day.
   • I want to give up _____ medication.
   • I want to live longer—and healthier.
   • I want to be in charge of my life.

5. Encourage yourself. When you're tempted to smoke, say to yourself, "I can put it off for five more minutes." When you successfully win over a temptation, say, "I made it." In the beginning, some people win only five-minute victories. No matter how small or seemingly trivial, whenever you overcome any desire to smoke, say to yourself, "Well done."

6. Speak positive, reinforcing messages to yourself several times each day. One victorious man said he divided his day into three sections. Each morning he would say, "I choose not to smoke before noon." At noon, he would say, "I choose not to smoke before I leave work." After work, he would say, "I choose not to smoke this evening."

   Even though he had moments of depression for the times he did give in, he determined to be kind to himself. "I forgive myself for failing. I choose not to smoke before noon today."

   By working in segments of time, he overcame his addiction. "I knew I could hold out for a few hours," he said. "I didn't know if I could hold out for a day or a week." The small victories reinforced his willpower and determination.

7. Begin an exercise program. As you rebuild your body, you will feel better, and your morale will increase. This will become a powerful weapon for you.

8. Enlist others to encourage you. Ask for help from your mate, a friend, a coworker. Join a self-help group such as Smokers Anonymous. Anyone who shares your desire for you to quit can strengthen you and make you realize that every minor victory *is* still a victory.

9. Free yourself from situational habits. Many people smoke in particular places, so

   • avoid crowds and other places where you normally light up
   • get rid of ashtrays in your home

- don't allow yourself to smoke when you drive
- get involved in activities that put you in smoke-free environments, such as a health spa, church, or volunteer organizations

10. Find oral substitutes. Drink six to eight glasses of water each day. This helps to flush the nicotine out of your system. Eat low-calorie foods. Try sugarless gum. Think of these as temporary helps to get you past your nicotine withdrawal. Although it would be best to quit without the crutch of nicotine patches, a report in the June 1994 *JAMA (Journal of the American Medical Association)* says these patches have doubled smokers' prospects of quitting successfully.

11. Don't give in to negative arguments. You may find yourself framing reasons for why you can't quit. When these thoughts come to you, answer them with positive information.

Here are examples:

- *I'll gain weight.* Answer: "Three to five extra pounds is worth the benefits I'll get through improved health." Or "I'll begin an exercise program to counteract the possible weight gain."

- *I've been smoking too long.* Answer: "It's not too late to quit. My body begins to rebuild as soon as I do."

- *I've failed before.* Answer: "Yes. But I won't fail this time. This time I'm committed to win the war."

- *My friends smoke.* Answer: "I'll avoid being around my friends when they smoke, or I'll ask them not to smoke around me. And I'll ask them, as my friends, not to offer me any cigarettes."

- *What's the difference? You have to die of something.* Answer: "I choose to die later and to live a healthier lifestyle. Smoking ages my body, and I want to live longer and healthier."

12. Pray for help. The Bible calls the body a temple (1 Cor. 3:16–17; 6:19). God will help you as you try to keep your "temple" clean and healthy.

Not smoking is one step I can take toward living ten years longer and healthier.

DOWN WITH FAT AND CHOLESTEROL

CHAPTER 10

HERE ARE three questions many people ask about cholesterol. Some of the answers may surprise you.

• • •

1. *Aren't fat and cholesterol really the same thing?* Although cholesterol and fat are often linked, they are different. Dietary cholesterol comes *only* from animal products. Plant-based food —vegetables, fruit, nuts, grains, and vegetable oils—contain no cholesterol. Both plant and animal products contain fat.

2. *Should I try to eliminate cholesterol completely?* Not if you want to stay alive. Cholesterol is essential to life. Among other things, it is used as a fatty insulation sheath around nerve fibers in the outer membrane of cells and as a building block for certain hormones. Your body manufactures plenty of cholesterol for your needs from the fat you get from plant-based foods.

3. *Do I need fat in my diet?* Yes. Since the early 1990s, the media has widely reported published medical research on the need for westerners to reduce their dietary fat intake. Some have taken this to mean that to be really healthy, they have to eliminate all fat. Not true. Your body needs a certain amount of fat, which is a concentrated energy source. It also provides essential fatty acids that help to absorb fat-soluble vitamins, make

food taste good, and give you a feeling of satisfaction when you have finished eating.

Once you ingest fat, your body *converts* fatty acids into substances that regulate many bodily processes, including normal cell growth, physical activity, and proper nerve functions. You must have the substances made from these essential fatty acids to

- maintain hormonal balance
- resist disease through your body's immune system
- lower blood pressure
- decrease the clumping of blood cells
- lower blood cholesterol

However, moderation is a key here, and the most healthful fat sources are plants. Research shows that more cancers develop as dietary fat intake increases from 10 to 40 percent of the calories consumed, especially if the fat comes from animal-based foods. Prostate cancer death rates as well as cancer of the testes, ovaries, uterus, breast, colon, and rectum correspond with high fat intake. In short, eating animal fat increases the risk of several cancers.

> If you are a typical American, 37 percent of your calories come from fat—more than twice what you need.
>
> The diets of most lacto-ovo vegetarians (those who use dairy products) consist of less than 20 percent fat. This helps account for their longer and healthier lives.

THE FACTS ABOUT CHOLESTEROL

Cholesterol is a white, waxy, fatlike substance. There are two different kinds of cholesterol, even though they are chemically the same.

One comes from food, called dietary cholesterol. You get this type only from eating animal products, such as meat and dairy products. The other kind is made by your body. Both end up in the blood.

When too much cholesterol is present in the blood, fatty deposits containing cholesterol build up along artery walls. This buildup narrows the blood vessels and restricts blood flow. When this process, known as atherosclerosis, occurs in an artery in the brain, the result can be a stroke. A blockage in the coronary arteries can cause angina (chest pains) or a heart attack.

The risk of heart disease rises with increasing levels of blood cholesterol although it doesn't rise markedly until levels exceed 200. Above 220, the rate of coronary heart disease begins to accelerate rapidly. Thus, many researchers urge you to keep your cholesterol levels as low as possible—preferably below 200. *You can do this through diet and exercise* (see Getting Practical).

Suppose you have had your cholesterol tested and the results show you are in a risk category for developing heart disease. In that case, quite likely your doctor will order a second blood test to measure the amount of HDL (High Density Lipoprotein) and LDL (Low Density Lipoprotein) cholesterol in your bloodstream. If your HDL (often called the "good" cholesterol) levels are low, you are more prone to develop arterial deposits—even if your total cholesterol level is below 200.

> LDL clogs arteries and increases the risk of heart disease.
> HDL removes cholesterol from cells.

The HDL level in an average adult American male ranges from 45 to 65. A woman's HDL range is usually higher. Studies suggest that you need a level above 70 to protect you against heart disease. Those below 35 are at coronary risk.

Genes and diet both influence your cholesterol levels. You can't alter your genetic heritage, but in most cases, a diet low in saturated fat and cholesterol will help you keep your blood cholesterol levels down.

Getting Practical

1. Begin to rid your diet of as much saturated fat from animal sources as possible. Replace butter with an olive oil spread, natural peanut butter, or margarine made from 100 percent corn, sunflower, or safflower oil. (We suggest that you avoid any margarine that includes hydrogenated fats.)

2. Substitute unsaturated fats for saturated. Polyunsaturated fats, such as safflower, flaxseed, and corn oil; and monounsaturated fats, such as olive oil, help to lower blood cholesterol levels. Monounsaturated fats may help you maintain or increase your HDL level. Use more foods that are high in omega-3 oils, such as flaxseed oil, nuts, wheat germ, soybeans, and avocados.

3. Lose weight if necessary. Not only does excess body fat raise your total blood cholesterol and LDL levels, but it is also an independent risk factor for heart disease. On average, for every two pounds of excess fat you carry, your body contributes 1 mg/dl of total cholesterol. At least one study says that when you lose weight, you get a 10 percent increase in HDL.

4. Get into an exercise program. Regular, aerobic exercise can help lower total cholesterol and raise HDL.

5. Eat more foods high in soluble fiber. Oat bran can lower cholesterol levels as much as 19 percent if eaten as part of a low-fat, low-cholesterol diet. Legumes, especially soybeans, are another excellent source of soluble fiber. There are others— such as black-eyed peas, kidney beans, carrots, split peas, corn, and prunes. Don't overlook sweet potatoes, zucchini, broccoli, bananas, apples, pears, and oranges. (No one can say exactly how much soluble fiber you need to eat each day.)

6. Don't smoke. Smoking increases total cholesterol and reduces HDL.

7. Eat nuts that grow on trees. (Peanuts grow underground and *do not* have omega-3 oils.)

Ponder this:

A bypass costs about $40,000.

"How much does it cost to switch to spaghetti and take a walk?"—Dr. Neal Bernard, George Washington University School of Medicine, Washington, D.C.

ROUGHING IT WITH FIBER

What is fiber? Once called roughage, it is the nondigestible cell walls of plant material. *Fiber occurs only in plant food.* Although there are several kinds of fiber, there are two basic types, and some plants contain both.

The first is water soluble (sometimes called *soft fiber*) and is found mostly in vegetables, seeds, brown rice, barley, oats, and oat bran. It increases the bulk of your stool by absorbing water and hurrying wastes through your system. Some compare this form to a sponge because it absorbs many times its own weight in water and swells up within the intestine.

The second type, insoluble (or *hard fiber*), is found in seeds, fruit, and legumes and binds to the cholesterol that the liver secretes into the intestine.

What does fiber do for my body? Good dietary fiber content prevents colon problems, from constipation and hemorrhoids to diverticulitis. Soluble fiber enables you to excrete cholesterol, leaving less of it to be absorbed into your bloodstream. It also forms gels, holds food in your stomach longer, and delays food absorption so that sugar goes more slowly into the bloodstream. You're left with a feeling of satiety and well-being.

Fiber has an amazing ability to lower blood cholesterol. You can lower your cholesterol as much as 30 percent by eating a cup (measured before cooking) of oat bran every day. One way to do this is to eat about half a cup of oat bran—which you can cook just like oatmeal—for breakfast. Then, later in the day, eat two bran muffins. Even if your blood cholesterol level is average, you can lower it as much as 3 percent by eating just half a cup of oat bran each day.

High-fiber foods take longer to eat because they require more chewing. Because they are less dense, they contain fewer calories—a definite plus for weight control.

Not all fiber works the same, however. For instance, wheat bran improves regularity, but it doesn't lower cholesterol. Oat bran and oatmeal lower cholesterol better than they improve regularity. The solution is to eat a variety of forms of fiber.

How Much Fiber?

So how much fiber do you need? No one knows for certain. It depends on the size of your digestive system. The larger you are, obviously the more you need. If you weigh 100 pounds, you probably need between 20 and 25 grams. At 150 pounds, the figure is roughly 30 to 35, and those who weigh 200 pounds need 40 to 45 grams. Most Americans only eat about 10 to 12 grams each day.

You don't need to start measuring and counting grams. Instead, eat a variety of cereals, grains, vegetables, and fruits. If you eat at least *four* servings of whole-grain bread and cereals and *five* fruits and vegetables each day, you will get your needed fiber intake. What could be easier?

Research suggests that 20 percent of Americans don't eat breakfast (unless we count a slice of toast or a Danish with coffee). Yet breakfast is an excellent time to get 6 or more grams of hard fiber from oat bran or cracked wheat cereal. About 30 percent of the population eat no fruit, or at most only a single serving a day. The same holds true regarding vegetables. And for too many, "salad" is the garnish that comes with a burger.

Getting Practical

1. Increase your fiber intake slowly, but consistently, to give your digestive system a chance to adjust. If you add it too quickly, you'll suffer from cramps, gas, bloating, or diarrhea.

2. Don't get too much of a good thing—follow the guidelines mentioned earlier. If you take in too much fiber, you may hamper mineral absorption.

3. As much as possible, eat the *skins* of fruits and vegetables.

4. The less processed a product is, the better it is for you. Manufacturers have refined many of our foods and, in so doing, have thrown out the fiber. White rice and white flour are good examples of highly refined foods. Opt instead for brown rice and whole wheat flour.

5. Form the habit of eating several vegetables and fruits at every meal.

6. Stress variety in your eating.

7. Drink six to eight glasses of water a day. Otherwise, fiber can slow down or block intestinal digestion.

8. Try to eat foods high in fiber at every meal.

ADD STARCHES TOO

"But potatoes make you fat," one woman insisted. "I never eat potatoes or rice."

She already had enough weight on her body to be labeled obese, but she still clung to a few "facts" she had learned somewhere along her diet journey. Even though she doesn't realize it, she needs starches, such as potatoes, bread, beans, and rice, to get complex carbohydrates.

What Are Carbohydrates?

Carbohydrates come almost exclusively from plant-based food—grains, fruit, vegetables, and the foods made from them, such as cereals and breads. All carbohydrates get broken down by the digestive tract and end up as glucose. Blood absorbs the glucose from the intestines, and the body uses it for energy. As you may have learned in school, we divide carbohydrates into two classes: simple and complex:

Simple refers to sugars (including glucose and fructose from fruits and vegetables, lactose from milk, and sucrose from cane or beet sugar).

Complex refers to starches as well as to cellulose or fiber, which occurs in all plant food.

What's the real difference between the two types of carbohydrates? Within minutes, simple sugars enter the bloodstream as glucose. This creates a rise in blood sugar and insulin. You feel great. But your body, in an attempt to balance itself, then reacts with an energy dip. If you have ever felt faint or shaky an hour or so after a heavy-sugar meal, that's the reason.

Complex carbohydrates (starches) take longer to digest. This means they don't elevate blood sugar as quickly. The high-fiber content of unrefined starchy foods also helps to even out the rate of digestion and absorption.

For better health, the answer is simple: Choose starches over refined sugars.

Getting Practical

1. Eat a wide variety of complex carbohydrates, which are found in vegetables and fruits, whole grains, and nuts.

2. Avoid simple sugars.

I want to live longer and healthier,
so I eat a variety of fruits, vegetables, and grains.

AVOIDING THE FIVE WORST DISEASES

"WHAT DO you people die of?" has become a common question to those who follow the Live-Longer Lifestyle.

. . .

"The same diseases as other people," we reply, "but not for another ten to fifteen years."

The bad news:

JAMA (Journal of the American Medical Association), reporting on its ten-year program to improve American health (Healthy People 2000), said that those with an average life span can expect to spend twelve unhealthy years coping with pneumonia, heart disease, cancer, diabetes, or disabilities caused by work-related injuries or violence.

Every day in the United States, about 2,700 people die from heart disease and 1,430 die from cancer. These deaths are largely unnecessary. Scientists have estimated that 60 percent of them are due to diet and a few other factors that individuals could control if they chose to.

This means that individuals—all of us—have numerous opportunities to cut down the number of these premature deaths.

Let's look at the top five catastrophic diseases and see how the health practices of those who follow the Live-Longer Lifestyle retard their onset.

1. HEART DISEASE

Heart disease in the Western world is so common that most people accept it as a normal part of life.

It is not a natural disease.

Your heart is a strong muscle, about the size of a fist. The pumping motion it makes as it sends blood throughout the body is measured as your heartbeat. On an average day, your heart beats about 100,000 times. Like any other muscle, the heart needs a continuous supply of oxygen and nutrients, which it gets from the blood that flows through the coronary arteries.

Blood vessels are designed to expand and contract as the heart pumps blood through them. If your arteries stay clean and flexible, your heart has an easy job. If they get clogged and hardened with deposits of fat and cholesterol, your heart must work harder to push blood through them. This also increases the pressure in the arteries. It's something like trying to send water through an ever-narrowing garden hose.

The progressive hardening and blocking of arteries by cholesterol and other substances is called atherosclerosis. This complex process probably starts when high levels of cholesterol in the bloodstream cause some type of damage to the artery wall. Fats, cholesterol, calcium, and other substances that are deposited and build up along the artery wall are known as plaque. Nicotine and high blood pressure can also damage arteries.

If one of your arteries becomes completely blocked, obviously blood can't flow through it. In coronary heart disease, the arteries supplying blood to the heart become blocked. The portion of your heart that doesn't receive enough oxygen eventually dies, and you have what we call a heart attack.

In Western countries, atherosclerosis generally gets worse as you age. However, during the Korean conflict, autopsies done on two thousand American soldiers—whose average age was twenty-two—revealed that 75 percent of them had already developed significant atherosclerosis. Since then, we have discovered the first stages of heart disease in children. About 45 percent of all heart-attack victims are younger than sixty-five. Most people haven't yet realized that most of the causes are diet related.

One piece of good news is that blood-cholesterol levels respond quickly to dietary change. Two dietary components—cholesterol, which is found only in animals and animal products, and saturated fat—increase LDL (bad) cholesterol. Decreasing your use of these products can lower your LDL levels.

Generally speaking, for every 1 percent reduction in your total blood-cholesterol levels, your risk of heart disease goes down 2 percent. Taking daily doses of vitamin E also appears to cut the risk of heart disease by one-third to one-half.

The Live-Longer Lifestyle studies, whose participants primarily eat a vegetarian diet, have confirmed such findings and have also shown the benefit of eating nuts. Peanuts and almonds are high in monounsaturated fat, walnuts are high in polyunsaturated fat, and both types are healthier than saturated fat. They also contain vitamin E, which reduces plaque buildup in the arteries.

"We found something we didn't really expect," said Dr. Gary Fraser, current head of the Adventists Health Study. "Those who ate nuts five or more times a week had only about half the risk of a fatal heart attack, as compared with those who ate nuts less than once a week." (This also applied to nonfatal heart attacks.)

Most people today know about the importance of low cholesterol and the beneficial effects of soluble fiber in reducing cholesterol levels. However, the cholesterol-and-fiber information is only a small part of what you need to know.

For instance, the *kind of protein* you eat also largely determines your risk for heart attack. One of the best ways to lower the blood cholesterol risk is to replace red meat with soy protein. You can find soy in such products as tofu, tempeh (made from whole cooked soybeans infused with a starter bacteria and allowed to ferment), soymilk, and miso (a soybean paste with salt, rice or barley, and a fermenting agent added). But it's not enough to just add soy to the diet. The whole diet matters, and a heart-healthy one should include soy, be low in saturated fat—and contain generous portions of food from plants.

2. CANCER

Cancer is on the increase throughout the United States and especially among baby boomers (those born between 1946 and 1965).

Even with all the cancer information available today, few people seem to realize that a low-fat, high-fiber diet can go a long way toward preventing various types. Although research continues to explain how this works, it is clear that diet is the single most important factor in helping the body fight the onset of cancer.

Several studies have indicated that a high-fat diet alone accounts for the high rate of breast cancer in the United States. Women who eat meat process estrogen differently from vegetarians. Apparently, meat-eaters recycle more of the estrogen and end up keeping more of it in their blood, while vegetarians pass more of it out of their bodies. Women vegetarians are less likely to develop breast cancer because they have less estrogen (which plays a key role in many breast cancers) in their bodies.

Reduce your risk of cancer by:

- building up your immunity with adequate rest, following sound principles of good health, and, especially, eating a good diet that includes whole grains and plenty of fruits and vegetables

- maintaining a sensible exercise program

- eating a lot of cruciferous vegetables, such as cabbage, broccoli, and cauliflower, and avoiding such substances as alcohol and tobacco

- cutting down (or eliminating!) caffeine

- getting rid of as much animal fat in your diet as you can

- keeping your weight within the normal range

- enjoying daily sunshine, but avoiding excessive exposure

- (for women) examining your breasts monthly and getting an annnual Pap smear

3. DIABETES

Does it surprise you to learn that of the thirty million diabetics in the world, slightly more than half live in the United States? This disease is hardly known in 80 percent of the world's population, which can't afford the fat-rich American diet. Worse, diabetes continues to increase in the West.

Diabetes occurs when the body becomes unable to handle glucose (sugar), which piles up to dangerous levels in the blood. There are two kinds and causes.

Type I Diabetes ("juvenile diabetes") accounts for about 10 percent of diabetics, whose bodies don't produce insulin. This disease is usually hereditary, although it can develop from viral infections. These people must take insulin to stay alive.

Type II Diabetes ("adult-onset diabetes") is officially called NIDDM—Non-Insulin Dependent Diabetes Mellitus—and afflicts about fifteen million Americans.

A typical high-fat diet combined with low fiber intake, middle age, and obesity (especially weight gain in the midsection) sets the stage for the development of adult-onset diabetes. These diabetics have too much glucose in their blood and urine and not enough in their cells—which need glucose for nourishment and to produce body energy. While their pancreases produce sufficient insulin, cells are unable to use it and it can't do its job properly.

After you eat, food is absorbed from your intestines into your blood, and part of it gets converted to glucose. Insulin, a pancreatic hormone, is a "chemical messenger" that signals the cells to "open up" and take in nourishment.

Microscopic pits in the cell walls, now being called *receptors,* unlock the cells and allow the glucose to enter. Insulin has to touch the receptors to activate them. If inadequate insulin reaches the cells, they can't take in the needed glucose. The cells starve while glucose piles up in the blood, spills over into the urine, and is finally eliminated.

The body recognizes that its cells are not getting enough glucose and signals the pancreas to produce more and more insulin. After years of working overtime, however, the pancreas stops—not because the pancreas is defective, but because of cellular insensitivity that relates to obesity and especially to a high fat intake. When cells have high fat levels, the glucose in the blood can't get into the cells.

However, a low-fat, more-natural diet and the resultant weight loss cause insulin receptors to become responsive to insulin once again and also increase the number of receptors.

Fiber also plays an important role in the control of diabetes. Fiber absorbs water in the digestive tract and creates a natural "sponge." When food particles become suspended in this spongy mass, they are more slowly absorbed into the bloodstream. This helps the body to keep blood sugar even. However, eating sugar and refined or fiberless food can cause a rapid rise in blood sugar levels. This activates the pancreas to release insulin to normalize the sudden glucose increase.

As diabetes progresses, most sufferers also develop severe problems: Diabetes is now the leading cause of blindness, and a high percentage of people with the disease have serious kidney damage. Diabetes also promotes atherosclerosis, more than doubles the risk of heart disease and stroke, and can lead to sexual impotence, gangrene, and hearing impairment.

Insulin injections, used for more than 70 years, and oral drugs, in use for the past 40 years, help to control the disease, but they do not cure it. There is no known medical cure for diabetes.

The Longevity Center in Santa Barbara found that many diabetics who followed low-fat, high-fiber diets and regular exercise programs were able to discontinue their daily insulin injections or substantially reduce their dosages. On a low-fat diet, the body's natural ability to produce insulin takes over, and it can stabilize on diet alone. Some doctors now say that at least 50 percent of diabetics—even if they have taken medication for years—can rid themselves of diabetes within months. (See page 200 for resources.)

4. HYPERTENSION

Hypertension is another word for high blood pressure—and it kills. About thirty-five million Americans have hypertension and another twenty-five million live on the edge of it.

Those with hypertension are three times more likely to have a heart attack and are eight times more likely to suffer a stroke than people with normal blood pressure. Hypertension is the single most significant factor in the half-million strokes suffered every year in the United States—and 150,000 of them cause death. Even among those people who do survive, a high percentage remain permanently limited by paralysis or speech and thought-pattern disturbances.

Hypertension can hit anyone at any age, but it's more common among those over age forty. In the United States, almost half of the population over forty have high blood pressure. Among those over sixty-five, the figure jumps to 70 percent.

How Blood Pressure Works

It takes a certain amount of pressure to push fresh, oxygenated blood through your body. Each time your heart contracts, about once a second, the blood pressure in your arteries increases. When your heart relaxes between contractions, the pressure decreases.

When you have your blood pressure taken, you get two readings. The higher reading (systolic) measures the pressure during contraction, while the lower (diastolic) measures the pressure between contractions. The National Institutes of Health defines *hypertension* as systolic pressure at or above 140 or diastolic pressure at or above 90.

For every ten points above a 140 systolic pressure, you increase the risk of heart disease or stroke by 30 percent. (This figure, of course, refers to persistent high readings; blood pressure varies from hour to hour.)

What causes hypertension? Researchers don't fully understand the cause of essential hypertension (about 90 percent of all hypertension cases; the other 10 percent have known causes, such as kidney disease or atherosclerosis). They have, however, defined four definite contributing factors—and three are diet related.

1. *Salt is the number one factor in hypertension.* By comparing Americans with people in other societies, we know that salt, not a cultural or racial factor, is the culprit. All the research shows that low-salt-using societies are low-blood-pressure societies. When people from low-salt-using societies enter Western nations and adopt Western dietary habits, their levels of hypertension increase. Within a short time, there is no difference between them and other westerners. The cure is simple: Cut down on the amount of salt ingested.

2. *Arterial plaque is the second most significant factor in hypertension.* Plaque infiltrates your blood supply lines, and fat and cholesterol attach themselves to the walls of your arteries and begin to harden. As plaque builds up and restricts the free flow of blood through the arteries, your blood pressure goes up as your heart works harder to get nutrients to your body. You can decrease blood pressure by eliminating excess fat and cholesterol from your diet and thus from your arteries.

3. *Obesity directly contributes to high blood pressure.* Fat needs to be fed. Every pound of fat in your body requires thousands of extra blood vessels. It takes more (i.e., higher) blood pressure to get blood through them. Obese people are five times more likely to have hypertension. Nearly everyone who is 20 percent overweight will eventually experience high blood pressure. Lose the weight to lower your risk.

> The accepted definitions of *overweight* and *obesity:* If you are 10 percent above your ideal weight, you are overweight; if you reach 20 percent, you are clinically labeled obese.

4. *Estrogen is an added danger for women.* A hormone used in birth control pills and to help women control the effects of menopause, estrogen is one cause of salt retention. To make it worse, estrogen also increases the production of angiotension, a substance that raises blood pressure and reduces blood flow to the kidneys—a dangerous combination. If you have questions about estrogen replacement, consult your physician.

You can stop high blood pressure, but not through taking diuretics (water pills), which have been the foundation of hypertension treatment for more than forty years. Diuretics force the kidneys to excrete abnormal amounts of salt and water. (Sometimes people take other drugs to blunt the side effects of the diuretics.) But antihypertensive drugs don't cure, they only control. Once people stop taking the pills, their blood pressure soars.

Here are four things you can do for yourself to reduce hypertension:

1. Reduce salt use.

2. Increase daily water intake to at least eight glasses.

3. Reduce dietary fat and excess weight.

4. Increase physical exercise.

5. OSTEOPOROSIS

The word *osteoporosis* probably conjures a visual image of stooped elderly people with weak bones.

Osteoporosis is a bone disease, not a disease of aging. It is a marginal nutritional deficiency (lack of calcium) that begins in young people. However, its effects don't usually show up until about age fifty.

Calcium deficiency begins to manifest in middle age as low-back pain, shorter stature, hunched shoulders. Women suffer from this more often than men. As the bones become less dense, they become weaker and more porous (*osteo* means bones and *porosis* means porous).

This disease causes bones to become so weak they shatter like glass and can't be repaired. Most experts believe that bones break and so people fall instead of the other way around. Although not fatal, the consequences of the broken bones are often so devastating that many elderly women never fully recover, and broken bones from osteoporosis are a leading cause of death in this segment of the population.

Yet osteoporosis is a preventable, treatable disease. You can prevent osteoporosis at any point along the way through sufficient dietary calcium and other needed nutrients along with strength-training exercises.

Modern medicine can do much to stop bone loss and improve bone density, but it always requires calcium. The foods with the highest level of calcium are collards, turnip greens, spinach, mustard greens, and broccoli. Hazelnuts and sunflower seeds are also high.

Women need to take 1,000 mg of calcium each day before menopause and increase it to 1,500 after menopause. You can get 1,000 mg of calcium by eating six flowerettes of broccoli. You also need to avoid items that increase calcium loss, such as an excess of caffeine, meat or other forms of protein, alcohol, and any use of tobacco.

Finally, your bones need exercise for strength. (Is this beginning to sound familiar?) "Use it or lose it" applies here. Exercise is important and you never outgrow the need for it.

Exercise, adequate calcium intake, plenty of rest, and sunlight (for vitamin D) can keep bones healthy.

GETTING PRACTICAL

Here are ten practical things anyone can do to live a healthier, longer life. Read them carefully, even though you've read them several times already in this book. They're worth repeating.

1. Stop smoking or using tobacco products. This includes exposure to second-hand smoke.

2. Begin and maintain a regular exercise program, such as walking for about half an hour three or four times a week.

3. Drink at least eight glasses of water every day.

4. Eat fruit—a lot of it—including at least three of these varieties daily: apples, pears, oranges, grapefruit, apricots, strawberries, cantaloupe, kiwi, papayas, bananas, dried figs. The fresher the fruit, the higher its nutritional value.

5. Eat more vegetables—including at least four vegetables a day, such as broccoli, cabbage, carrots, sweet potatoes, spinach, green peppers, cauliflower, peas, onions, lettuce, potatoes, tomatoes, radishes, and mushrooms.

6. Eat legumes three or four times a week. Choose from soybeans or soybean products, lentils, garbanzos, and just about any other kind of beans, fresh or dried.

7. When you fry, use olive or peanut oil; when you bake use vegetable oil instead of margarine or Crisco. In salads opt for

olive, linseed, or flaxseed oils because they're extremely high in omega-3 fats, which are low in American diets.

8. Eat a variety of whole grains and nuts. Choose brown rice instead of white rice. Include barley in your diet. Eat a variety of nuts such as almonds and walnuts.

9. Cut down on or avoid salt.

10. Reduce your intake of sugar. Especially watch for hidden sugars by reading ingredients on every food item you buy.

I will live longer and healthier if
I put off the worst diseases—and I can.

LOSE WEIGHT—FOREVER—WITHOUT DIETING

QUICK! IN the next ten seconds, name all the diets you have ever heard about. Remember the Scarsdale Diet? The Los Angeles Diet? The banana diet? Ever heard of the vinegar diet (a teaspoon of apple cider vinegar with every meal), or the low-carbohydrate, high-protein diet? How about the citrus diet? The rotation diet? Chances are you've tried a few of these yourself.

• • •

Here are a few revealing statistics: More than 80 million Americans are overweight—that means one out of three. They carry a total of 2.3 billion pounds of excess body fat. Estimates say that nearly 65 million people attempt to diet at least once during each year. Americans spend about 40 billion dollars annually to burn or sweat off pounds, reshape their bodies, or diet.

Don't think weight is just a problem for adults. New studies say that at least one in five children in the United States are obese. Lack of physical activity is an important contributor, and the weight problem appears to be getting worse.

You may be one of those trying to lose that excess body fat. If you have taken part in more than one program, you should know first-hand that diet failure isn't totally a lack of willpower. Instead, you may have put too much effort into the wrong methods. Do the following statements sound familiar to you?

"I have to monitor every calorie if I'm going to keep off those thirty-five pounds." Rigid calorie restriction is not necessary. It's not an enjoyable lifestyle because it's based on self-deprivation.

"If only I were a little more self-disciplined, I'd get the pounds off and keep them off." You do not have a weak character, and weight loss is not just a matter of discipline. No one can stay on a rigid diet indefinitely anyway. Only about 5 percent of those who diet manage to keep the weight off permanently. When diet is combined with behavior modification, that figure rises to 10 percent—but that's still low.

From past experience, you probably already know you can't maintain any diet that keeps you hungry. One of your most powerful instincts is to avoid starvation. The only diet you or anyone else can sustain is one that promotes weight loss and good health *and* that allows you to eat until you are full.

You formed bad eating habits over a lifetime, not just during the time it took to put on that extra 10 or 20 pounds. Your weight came on slowly, and you'll be more successful if you take it off slowly. The mind adjusts to weight loss much more slowly than the body does. While you may lose some weight fairly quickly, it takes time to adjust your mental image of your protruding stomach. I once heard someone say, "The fat leaves the body, but it takes longer for the fat to leave the head."

If you expect to find a magic method that will leave you thin for life, one that requires no effort and no self-discipline, you will fail. There is no magic method. Losing weight is a complex problem that presents a challenge to those who truly want to shed excess pounds.

Although we can't offer a magic formula, we can share the successful program that those in the Live-Longer Lifestyle group use—many for their entire lives. It's a fairly simple program, but it requires two things: (1) some self-discipline and (2) sufficient time to work. You won't find this an instant weight-loss program. But take heart. If you lose weight quickly, you are three times more likely to regain it than if you lose weight slowly.

The eating program prescribed by the Live-Longer Lifestyle says that you can learn how to eat to the feeling of satisfaction *without* counting calories or using tricks, such as substituting fat grams. You can eat an incredible variety of delicious food and still lose excess pounds. When you do, you'll join hundreds of thousands of others who already know success.

Here are two important points to keep in mind when you start a long-term weight-loss program:

1. Long-term, gradual loss offers more permanent results. You are less likely to regain the weight.

2. A moderate weight-loss program puts less stress on your body. Quick-loss programs, especially unhealthy ones, can hasten the aging process.

If you lose weight through drastic reductions in caloric intake alone, you haven't solved any problems. Such diets may work—temporarily—but they aren't a *lifestyle* you can follow indefinitely. The more healthful kind of weight loss involves learning to eat properly. Would you really want to go on day after day at a near-starvation level? Could you stick with such a program indefinitely? By trying such methods, you may set yourself up for severe health problems in the future.

Low-calorie dieting disrupts your body's metabolism. When you start a restricted diet, your body thinks it's starving. Consequently, your metabolism slows down. God created us with this response to avoid starvation.

If you have dieted several times, you know that you lose most of your weight during the first weeks. You've probably known the ecstasy of losing five or ten pounds in a week. But by the fourth week or so, you can't seem to drop a single ounce. You see, once your body starts to slow down, it fights against weight loss.

Regular dieters speak of reaching plateaus. "I can lose the first ten pounds with almost no effort," said Valerie, "then I'm stuck. I can't seem to get any lower." She didn't realize it, but each time she dieted, she fought against her own body. Once the cycle of weight loss kicks in, *your metabolism slows for as long as two months, even after you start eating normally again.*

Until the late 1980s, almost all weight-loss programs had a simple, two-prong approach: (1) Cut total caloric intake and (2) exercise. Such programs are somewhat effective and for some people have been enough.

Research shows that for most people, however, simple caloric restriction, even with the addition of an exercise program, isn't the answer. They may drop the extra pounds, but they haven't done anything to enhance their health.

Part of the problem is the popular notion that a calorie is a calorie. Therefore, if you cut calories, you cut weight.

But this is only partially true.

To control weight *and* embrace a healthy lifestyle, you need to make changes you can live with for the rest of your life. You can't do this if you attempt to go on day by day without satisfying your hunger. You need a lifestyle that will do four things for you:

1. Satisfy your hunger and leave you feeling full.
2. Incorporate foods that encourage better health while helping you lose weight.
3. Help you to stop storing fat in your body.
4. Burn the fat.

Now let's look at the Live-Longer Lifestyle solution.

Please read the following statement at least twice because you may not want to believe it.

> Complex carbohydrate and plant-based protein calories—even if taken in excess—are seldom converted and stored as fat.

If you grasp that simple statement—which is easily verified—you are on your way to a healthier lifestyle *and* permanent weight loss.

Look at it this way. By nature, your body is efficient at storing *fat* calories. You use only about 3 percent of the calories in fat to digest, transport, and deposit it into your body's fat storage areas. However, your body metabolizes protein calories and excretes the by-products rapidly. Excess protein can create other problems, of course; it can stress your liver and kidneys by forcing them to work overtime. But excess protein doesn't usually add to obesity. *You have no efficient metabolic pathway in your body by which you can turn protein into fat for storage.*

You rarely store carbohydrates as fat, *even when you eat to excess.* Surprised at that?

For years, you've probably heard that potatoes are fattening, but that simply is not true. (It is true, however, that the fat-laden butter and sour cream often added to potatoes are fattening.) The metabolic pathways that your body uses to convert extra carbohydrates into fat and then store them take 24 percent of the calories found in carbohydrates. This is a highly inefficient use of the energy in carbohydrates, which means there's less to store. Of course, the closer the food is to its natural state, the better and more healthful.

In studies where researchers put radioactive markers for carbohydrates in food, they learned that *less than 1 percent* of the carbohydrate load was converted into fat and stored. Even when people ate carbohydrates excessively, they generally burned them up in "wasteful" metabolic creations that tend to increase the body's metabolic rate—not reduce it, as happens in calorie-restricted diets.

A note of caution:

All oils are 100 percent fat, even olive oil. At room temperature oils are liquid. Every one of them contains 9 calories per gram. Fat is the most calorically dense food in nature.

Your body treats all fats as reserve fuel and stores it, mostly under the skin surface and around organs, in case you have insufficient carbohydrate intake in the future.

The side benefit of following the Live-Longer Lifestyle in losing weight is that it will keep you trim, strong, and healthy. The weight-loss suggestions given here are a safe and healthy way of living you can follow for the rest of your now-longer life span. (Note: If you are seriously ill, please consult a doctor who understands nutrition before you make any significant changes in your diet.)

GETTING PRACTICAL

1. Write down your goals—for weight loss, better heath, and better eating habits—and review your goals regularly, say once a week.

2. Forgive yourself when you fail. Nobody is perfect. If you fail, admit it to yourself and say, "I will do better." Don't let one temporary lapse become a permanent failure.

3. Get support. Research suggests that if your mate or a close friend offers *positive* verbal support (this does not include reprimands for lapses), you have a greater chance for success. Positive reinforcement encourages the continuation of good behavior.

4. Reward yourself with extra time to relax or a small present—anything that's personally meaningful to you—for sticking with your plan. Do not use food as a reward.

5. Start the day with a big breakfast and have a small lunch and supper. Or you might go on a two-meal-a-day plan. Include several types of fruit and vegetables.

6. Don't snack between meals. When you finish your evening meal, make it the final bit of food that goes into your body until breakfast. Maintaining the water-drinking habit will help depress your appetite.

7. Begin meals with food that contains both protein and fat. Your appetite control system needs these two ingredients before the appetite begins to slow.

Try starting your meals with soup. A study done by Dr. Henry Jordan of the University of Pennsylvania showed that those who started lunch or dinner with a bowl of soup ate 54.5 fewer calories each meal. Some researchers suggest saving salad and fruit until after the main course of fat and protein.

8. Don't put more food on the table than you expect to eat at that meal. For most people, seeing an abundance of food on the table creates a desire to eat more than they need. Alternatively, put all the food on the table, serve, and immediately remove all leftovers from the table.

9. Remind yourself to eat slowly. Chew thoroughly and slowly. Put your fork down between bites. Eating too fast causes some overweight people to eat too much. No matter how much food you eat, it takes your brain about 20 minutes to recognize that you have eaten enough to satisfy your body's needs.

10. Need dessert to finish the meal? This is a learned behavior, and you can change it. If you eat salad or fruit at the end of the meal, you may actually solve your problem.

11. Leave the table as soon as you have finished your meal and start some kind of activity—doing dishes, walking, or light gardening. If others are at the table and you want to continue to talk, take away your own plate, and return to the table.

12. When you leave the table feeling full but not stuffed, tell yourself, "This is the way I'm supposed to feel. I am satisfied, but I'm not stuffed."

I want to live healthier and longer,
so I will maintain a healthy weight.

READING FOOD LABELS

Since 1994, the Food and Drug Administration has required food manufacturers to display nutritional labels on most foods. These "Nutritional Facts" contain several items of information for weight-conscious people.

Nutrition Facts	
Serving Size: 1/2 cup dry (40g)	
Servings Per Container 13	
Amount Per Serving	
Calories 150	
Calories from Fat	25
	% Daily Value*
Total Fat 3g	**5%**
Saturated Fat 0.5g	2%
Polyunsaturated Fat 1g	
Monounsaturated Fat 1g	
Cholesterol 0mg	0%
Sodium 0mg	0%
Total Carb 27g	9%
Dietary Fiber 4g	15%
Soluble Fiber 2g	
Insoluble Fiber 2g	
Sugars 1g	
Protein 5g	
Vitamin A	0%
Vitamin C	0%
Calcium	0%
Iron	10%

* Percent Daily Values are based on a 2000 calorie diet. Your daily values may be higher or lower depending on your calorie needs.

- *Serving size.* Be aware: Manufacturers often place low, unrealistic serving sizes on their product labels —often the amounts are smaller than the average person eats. Notice that the higher the calories and fat in a product, the smaller the serving size listed on the label.

- *Calories.* Although counting calories is not as important to healthful weight loss as watching your fat intake, it's useful to know the number of calories in a serving. As a general rule, you're better off eating food with a lower number of calories and a larger serving size. This combination means it's also low in fat.

- *Calories from fat.* This number indicates the total fat calories in each serving size and includes all types of fat in the product.

To figure out the percentage of calories from fat in a product, divide the number of calories from fat by the total calories listed in the serving size. Multiply the result by 100 to obtain the percentage. A good rule of thumb is to avoid foods that get more than 27 percent of their calories from fat (generally, more than 3 grams of fat per 100 calories).

- *Percent Daily Value* can be misleading because it is based on a diet of 2,000 calories, and not everyone needs that many calories.

- *Total fat (listed in grams)*. Manufacturers break fat down according to its type, such as saturated or polyunsaturated. Avoid foods with a high level of saturated fats.

The rest of the label provides information about the product's cholesterol, sodium, potassium, total carbohydrates (including dietary fiber and sugar), protein, and vitamins and minerals.

Concentrate on three key elements: serving size, calories, and calories from fat. The total fat can help you keep track of how many grams of fat you eat each day.

Food-Label Terminology

- Fat-Free   fewer than .5 grams of fat per serving
- Low-Fat   3 or fewer grams of fat per serving
- Lean   fewer than 10 grams of fat per serving (can have as many as 89 calories)
- Light/Lite   1/3 fewer calories or no more than 1/2 the fat of the "regular" higher-calorie, higher-fat version (this may still be a lot

of fat); or no more than 1/2 the sodium
of the "regular" higher-sodium version
(this doesn't take fat into account)

- Cholesterol-Free   fewer than 2 mg of cholesterol and 2 or
fewer grams of saturated fat per serving
(this may still contain a lot of unsaturated fat from vegetable oils)

In summary, to maintain a reasonable weight, follow a simple lifestyle program. Remind yourself that you have control over your health as well as over the factors involved in permanent weight loss. You can maintain this by

- keeping up your water-drinking schedule
- being moderate in what, how much, and how frequently you eat
- staying with a regular walking program (or other form of exercise)
- slowing down your eating
- living in a positive atmosphere and with a positive attitude

Choosing the moderate approach described in this chapter should provide lasting results. Try the Live-Longer Lifestyle for at least three weeks and experience a noticeable improvement in your health.

Contrary to what some say regarding your part in this process, the primary decision to maintain your weight and health is your will and your desire to be in control of your life.

MORE THAN JUST FOOD

"I'M HUNGRY," your five-year-old child wails. "I want something to eat."

• • •

"But you just ate an hour ago," you reply.

"I'm hungry *now*," your child insists.

What do you do? If you're a typical parent, you decide it's easier to give your child a quick snack than to argue. And since you're an enlightened parent, you naturally offer a low-calorie, low-fat snack.

Was that the best thing for your child?

Just reading that question may surprise many. Most nutritionists prescribe three meals *plus* two snacks a day. Ever hear any experts prescribe a "sensible diet" that didn't allow for snacks? Snacking is part of living the Western lifestyle.

Did you know?

A 1970 study showed that 30 percent of the food Americans consumed came in the form of snacks. It's probably much higher today!

Eating between meals is a habit that Live-Longer Lifestyle nutritionists have been among the first to frown on. A major reason is that snacking usually doesn't provide any useful or nutritional function. Worse, snacking may actually harm the human body.

Consider the words *hunger* and *appetite.* True hunger has a physical basis, although most of us have said, "I feel hungry," as we reached for something to ingest—even when we knew we weren't hungry. We were, in fact, responding to our *appetite,* which is a desire, a yearning created in the mind. Appetite is a learned response. We also know that many people eat to satisfy emotional needs.

Your body has natural rhythms. One of those rhythms occurs in the digestive system. *Every time you snack, you interrupt the digestive process.*

This was shown in an experiment, which has been replicated many times, involving five people. Each of the participants ate a normal breakfast. It took them an average of 4 1/2 hours to empty their stomachs. A few days later, those five people ate a breakfast identical to the one eaten the first day. The researchers then introduced some variables.

1. One person ate an ice cream cone 2 hours after breakfast. The ice cream eater needed 6 hours to fully digest breakfast.

2. Three of the subjects snacked every half-hour after breakfast but ate no lunch. Their snacks consisted of a peanut butter sandwich, a piece of pumpkin pie with a glass of milk, and a half slice of buttered bread. After 9 hours, *they still had undigested breakfast foods in their stomachs.*

3. The fifth person ate two chocolate candy bars between breakfast and lunch and two more between lunch and dinner. In this case, *more than half of the breakfast remained in the stomach after 13 1/2 hours, as well as portions from the other meals eaten.*

Whenever you eat *anything,* you activate the digestive juices that aid in breaking down food. If you put new food into your stomach several hours into the digestion of the first meal, the stomach slows its work as it begins to process the new food. If you snack all day, your exhausted stomach will not get a chance to rest until late into the night.

Logic says that if your eating habits fatigue and weaken the digestive system, that weakening—even if you don't feel it physically—will extend to other parts of your body. That's reason enough to avoid snacking.

That's why we say, "Avoid snacking to give your stomach a chance to rest."

Note: If you have young children, it's important to give them meals at regular times. They may not be able to eat a large quantity at one time, so they may become painfully hungry before the next meal. You may choose to feed them earlier in the evening, such as shortly after school, rather than waiting until the family eats.

Above all, avoid rigidity with children regarding snacking. In the interest of kindness and consideration, you may need to compromise a bit until your children are a little older.

GRAZING

Experiments have shown that some people can graze and not gain weight. (Grazing refers to eating throughout the day, imitating such animals as cows.) This works as long as these people remember that grazing must be done in small amounts. As one woman said, "You have to live on the edge of hunger. You never eat enough at any one time to feel really full. You always aim to take in just a little each time." But grazing for weight control seldom works as an ongoing lifestyle.

Dr. John A. Scharffenberg, a Harvard-trained nutritionist at Loma Linda University, offers six reasons to avoid grazing:

1. Scientists have shown that demineralization (the destruction of the crystal framework of the tooth's surface) occurs for two hours after you begin to eat. Continual eating keeps demineralization

going all the time if you don't brush your teeth. This increases your risk of tooth decay.

2. Blood tryglycerides go up as soon as you start eating. Some snacks—such as sweets—make your platelets become sticky, and this increases clotting and the risk of heart attack.

3. Your blood sugar goes up as you eat, and that stimulates a need for more insulin. Continuous stimulation causes hyper-insulinism and increases your risk of a heart attack.

4. Digesting three large meals burns about 40 calories a day more than digesting the same amount of food consumed in smaller portions. This has implications for weight management.

5. Grazing can easily cause a preoccupation with food. This is especially true if you don't ever eat to a feeling of satisfaction. The act of snacking can easily lead to overindulgence.

   Eating can involve more than feeding a physical need. It can also become a conflict-resolution tool. By indulging and grazing, many people can temporarily overcome emotional traumas, such as loneliness, anger, or the need to feel loved. Afterward, however, there may be a struggle with guilt over the indulgence.

6. Grazing can cause other problems. For example, it can deplete hydrochloric acid, one of the two major protein-digesting enzymes in the stomach. If you snack regularly, it can disturb your sleep. And snacking on empty calories can result in malnutrition. Frequent snacking on such foods decreases your mental and physical efficiency.

   If you believe the media ads, commercial snack foods do just the opposite. Manufacturers are constantly urging you to try their products for a "quick picker-upper" or "to lose that run-down feeling." Candies, especially, get pushed as providers of quick energy.

   The truth is just the opposite. When you eat, your blood

flows from the muscles and brain to the digestive organs. Snacking disrupts this regular rhythm and interrupts your digestion of food. You can then end up with gas or heartburn.

LET'S LOOK AT BREAKFAST

Ever wonder why the morning meal is called breakfast? It literally means "break the fast," that is, to eat after having fasted for 9 to 12 hours.

> Here's the most important thing to remember
> about breakfast: *Eat it.*

Dozens of research projects have shown clearly that irritability and inattentiveness in youngsters directly relates to not eating a hearty breakfast. Many schools attempt to correct this problem by providing breakfast for students.

Adults who don't eat breakfast before going to work more easily become fatigued. Many grab snacks, including coffee or another caffeine source, to boost their energy. Research shows that these people generally have a reduced output and are more prone to accidents.

"But I just can't eat in the mornings," you may complain. "I'm just not hungry." That's probably because you do something wrong the night before. Do you go to bed late? If so, it may take a couple of hours to work up a good appetite the following morning. Try getting up earlier and exercising first.

Do you eat too much too late in the day? Do you have a late-night snack after a big evening meal? Do you spend your evenings reading or watching TV, activities that require little energy? If you do, your digestive process probably isn't complete before bedtime. Your stomach, small and large intestines, liver, and gall bladder have to keep on working into the night—and working with less efficiency. All your systems slow down during sleep, but they can't rest until they finish their work. Your digestive organs need rest as much as your muscles and brain. Consequently, in the morning, your digestive system is exhausted and you're bleary-eyed. The thought of food may even nauseate you for the first couple of hours you're awake. Now you understand why.

If you make your evening meal the lightest meal of the day, you will be ready to eat in the morning. When you eat a large, nutritious breakfast, your need for food intake decreases throughout the day. Eating a good breakfast is important in the battle against snacking.

In the 1980s hypoglycemia (low blood sugar) became a favored disease, and suddenly everyone had it. People suffered from fatigue and sometimes dizziness or fainting spells. The prescribed cure: Eat every 2 or 3 hours. Sometimes they were told to eat three normal meals with a snack in between meals. That is, they were told that snacking was good for them. The prescribers did nothing to figure out *why* patients felt fatigued or experienced other debilitating symptoms. They looked only for something to overcome the effects.

This is exactly what most snackers do—look for a way to get through the downtime most people feel in the afternoons. They use snacks to give them the pickup to make it through those late afternoon lows. When they undergo a noticeable drop in blood sugar and an increase in irritability or fatigue, their quick, easy response is a cup of coffee or a candy bar. Within minutes, their sagging spirits swing upward.

Let's look at that low time again. First, if you eat three solid meals a day, especially starting the day with a good breakfast, you can cure the worst of those low times.

If you're an average American, however, you have a compulsion to feel good all the time. That means you reach for a pill, a drink, or something to boost yourself when your energy level begins to drain. You want to keep your engines roaring at full blast from morning until night. If you start to "come down," you reach for a quick fix to get yourself back to "normal" again. But such lows are actually the wisdom of your body speaking to you; you just aren't listening.

If you're one of those who have gotten into the habit of snacking for a quick energy boost, you probably don't even realize what has been going on with your body. You are continually stressing your body with additional work during most of your waking hours. If your ultimate goal is to have the greatest energy, health, and sense of well-being possible, then quick fixes from refined snacks aren't the answer.

For those who want to live a healthier decade longer, this is one of those little-known but significant factors. It's simple: Eat nothing between meals. This is the time to drink water or, if you must, juice. Cold water curbs the appetite better than warm or hot.

A study conducted in Alameda County (California) followed its subjects over a nine-year period. It showed that the death rate for men who regularly snacked between meals *was 20 percent higher than for men who did not.*

GETTING PRACTICAL

If you want to become victorious over snacking and improve your digestion, here are five simple things you can do.

1. Make a commitment to stop snacking. Don't tell yourself, "I'll try." Think about it until you finally say, "I commit myself to snack-free living." Don't think, *I'll give up snacks.* To give up anything implies depriving yourself. Then this practice becomes no better than a diet. You are not giving up anything beneficial. You are moving toward more positive health.

2. Each day, eat a full breakfast, lunch, and dinner. Plan your meals around complex carbohydrates with a lot of grain, fruits, and vegetables.

3. If you feel the need to snack, drink a large glass of water instead. Flavor it with lemon or lime. Or try an unsweetened herbal tea. If you have eaten healthful meals, you won't need food between them. It will take time to establish the habit of reaching for water instead of potato chips, but you can do it. If you do fail one day, you have failed only that one day. You can start over again the next morning.

4. Learn to say, "No, thank you." American culture seems built around food. It's either a meal or a brunch or a dessert supper. When you are in a situation where someone offers you a snack, the simplest way to decline is to say, "No, thank you."

   Another possibility is to take the food for later, if it's convenient to do so, and say, "Thanks. When I eat my next meal, I'll include this."

5. Decide which three snack foods you have the most problem resisting. Let's say you have decided they are (1) chocolate ice cream, (2) Oreo cookies, and (3) buttered popcorn.

   Before you do anything else, remind yourself that you acquired these food preferences. You can cut back on them or eliminate them by substituting other, more healthful foods into your eating plan. Your goal is to train yourself to prefer food that you can eat with your meal and that you will enjoy.

   Begin with your third choice, the buttered popcorn. Go back to step 1 and commit yourself either to including a small portion of it as part of a regular meal, or cutting it from your life. Then, concentrate on cutting back or eliminating buttered popcorn.

   As you concentrate on this item, continue to remind yourself that you are striving for better health. Each time you succeed, compliment yourself by saying, "I have done a good job. I have a strong desire for good health." (You may ask health-minded friends to encourage you as well.)

Drinking a glass of water is one sensible way to fight temptation.

Once you have conquered the buttered popcorn, go on to Oreo cookies, then perhaps to chocolate ice cream.

A final word:

Snacking isn't a major factor in your overall health, as ingesting too much fat or not exercising enough is, but if you overcome the psychological objection to not snacking and decide to give your digestive system a needed rest, you will notice a difference in your energy level. Race horses don't race every day. In baseball, pitchers don't play every game. They value rest, and perhaps you should consider the same for your digestive system.

If you become successful with one of the smaller health practices, it can give you confidence to become successful in one of the more important health practices. Choosing not to snack provides you with an opportunity to demonstrate that you are in charge of your health.

Because I choose long life and excellent health,
I choose not to snack.

IT CAN KILL YOU!

CHAPTER 14

STRESS HEADACHES. Tension backaches. The TV ads subtly remind you that you live in a stress-filled world and you need to keep your medicine bottles handy.

• • •

They also tell you exactly which over-the-counter medications to buy. That's bad enough, of course, but despite all the research and knowledge you've accumulated about stress reduction and management, TV ads, medical journals, and popular entertainment continue to shout: "You still don't know how to cope with the stress!" The enormous sales of such prescription drugs as Prozac and Valium testify to the ongoing pressures of daily life.

PERCEPTION OF STRESS

Stress itself won't kill you, but not perceiving it or adapting to stressful situations can. You get into trouble when you deny or ignore the tensions in your life. However, if you're open to perceiving your personal stress, you have taken the first step toward coping.

The forces that cause stress usually confront us from without. Yet about 90 percent of the distress people experience stems from their negative *perceptions* of these forces. Reacting to stress with a view conditioned by a healthy philosophy can allow you to convert even critical stress into steppingstones of achievement.

So, how you perceive events is the key to stress management. (Of course, there are many good types of stress. Most people would consider milestone events, such as getting married, starting a dream job, graduating from college, or buying a home as positive, if stressful, experiences.)

Too often we don't recognize stress until it becomes extreme. We excuse it or name it something else, such as "seasonal work pressures" or "temporary tiredness." Some people have difficulty admitting they suffer from stress. You'll hear them say things like: "Maybe I'm a little tired, but I've been working long hours. Nothing to get concerned about. I'll be fine in a few days."

Nevertheless, stress has a way of identifying the weakest part of the body. Think about a metal chain; if you put extreme pressure on the chain, it will eventually snap at its weakest link. Your body responds the same way under the constant input of stress. You "snap" at your weakest part. In most people, this means the onset of physical problems.

All demands in life involve some tension, and stress remains a necessary ingredient of life. It's an expression of your lifelong experience with the *physical, psychological, social,* and *spiritual* demands of living.

Physical stress comes when your body gets out of balance. Too little or too much of anything can be a stressor. On the job, for instance, in an environment that places increased demands on you, your body may pay the price—especially if you resist your stressors. You may become physically unbalanced by too much adrenaline or too little of a particular kind of hormone. If you stay at the job long enough, eventually the ulcer, the heart attack, or some other stress-related illness will come along. Whenever you upset your delicate body harmony and keep it unbalanced for a prolonged period, your body rebels. For some, physical distress is the only way to get off the treadmill and get their lives into balance. Yet too many of us have not learned to listen to our bodies.

Psychological or mental stress arises primarily from the perception that you are not in control of a situation. Often people use the wrong coping methods in their attempts to regain control. They may turn to alcohol to relax or caffeine for energy. Some researchers believe that mental illness (including organic depression) may be the body's escape mechanism from too much mental distress.

Social stress arises from relationships with a spouse, family, friends, coworkers, or neighbors. If you're feeling intense pressure in the social realm, it overflows to other parts of your life.

Spiritual stress can be recognized as a decrease in spiritual fervor. "I used to go to church every week, and I know I ought to go now, but I just don't have the energy." Haven't most of you heard such statements? Perhaps you've even said them. That oblique reference to energy may be a telling message about the spiritual pressure in life.

Stress is subjective. Some stressors are universal. Life-threatening events, such as tornadoes, earthquakes, or serious illnesses, cause distress for almost anyone who experiences them.

Stress affects individuals in different ways. What makes you feel pressured and tense may be seen as an exciting challenge by another.

In a research project done from 1994 to 1996 at Wellesley College Center for Research on Women, Rosalind Barnett surveyed three hundred women in dual-career couples. She concluded that the more roles men or women had, the better they rated their own mental health. For them, what predicted stress wasn't the number of responsibilities they faced, but whether they found satisfaction from their spheres of life.

This doesn't contradict the fact that many people feel stressed when trying to do more things than they can realistically accomplish.

One way to look at stress is to think of it as the result of a misfit. Stress builds when you feel uncomfortable, unwanted, overwhelmed, or fearful. When you don't fit into your environment, tension results. To eliminate or minimize pressure, scrutinize your living or work space. Does it restrict you? Does it prevent a normal flow of energy? Perhaps you need to redesign it or move out of it.

To be free of stress, you need to live in an environment that fits you. This may mean you need to change jobs. Why be imprisoned in a vocation of drudgery? This isn't said to encourage sloth or drifting, but to encourage a reevaluation of your environment.

COMBATING STRESS

You may need to carefully examine your life and change the stress level you live in. You may need to get professional help regarding personal relationships. You may need to find a more emotionally supportive social group or church family. Or you may find ways to adapt to your current situations. Adaptation isn't merely giving in or conforming. It's grappling with problematic situations and learning from them—and finding different ways to approach them.

For instance, a year after Barbara became a reservationist for Delta Airlines, she complained that it was the most stressful job she had ever held. She didn't consider it possible to transfer. She liked the company and dealing with the public—most of the time. "But then, why do I feel so stressed?" she asked.

After several sessions with her pastor, she figured out ways to ward off the stress. For example, when customers became irate, she would say to herself, *This person isn't angry at me. She has a problem, and I'm the one she's taking it out on.* By constantly reminding herself of such things throughout the day, Barbara decreased her stress level.

"When customers dumped their anger or dissatisfaction on me," she said, "the tension headaches began. Slowly I began to acknowledge that even though I couldn't control everything about my work, I could control some things. When tension got to the blow-up level, I would say to myself, 'This is only a job. It's not my life.' And that helped."

Stress is always present, and it takes its toll. The combination of low control and high demands raises the risk for heart disease and other stress-related diseases. For example, cooks, waiters, cashiers, and assembly-line workers have higher rates of heart disease than those who feel they have a certain amount of control over their jobs.

People who live near airports and get daily noise blastings have higher rates of hypertension, heart disease, and suicide than the rest of the population. The stress of poverty and ghetto life in low-income neighborhoods causes hypertension in residents nearly twice as often as in those who live in less-crowded, lower-crime-rate neighborhoods with lower unemployment figures.

When you're young, you begin with high physical energy, but low psychological energy levels. As you go through life, your physical stamina decreases. If you had healthy parenting and developed positive experiences, your psychological energy increased. That is, you learned to adjust to the world you lived in and stayed in balance more easily.

You can liken your physical energy level to a large savings account that you live off your entire life. With time and usage, the balance begins to diminish as you face burdens and challenges. (But you can do things to slow its diminishing rate.)

In contrast, think of your psychological energy level as a checking account. While it may increase during your life, it also fluctuates more. You increase it when you receive a much-wanted promotion, become happily married, have a number of close friends, build or buy a home, go on a dream vacation, or have children who turn out to be credits to society. But this energy level also decreases considerably if you lose your job, face a difficult divorce, lose a home in a fire, or learn that your children are involved with drugs.

Your reaction to stress depends on you individually—on your vital force, which is created by combining your physical and psychological energies. How these two energy sources produce such a vital force isn't entirely clear, but we know that the more you have of both, the better your ability to cope with stress. That is, you can cope better with physical challenges as well as psychological or creative challenges.

Using this model of stress, you can see that your diet, exercise, whether you smoke or are overweight, and whether you are able to relax affect your physical energy savings account. Your sense of self-worth, attitudes, good deeds, and especially your spiritual values, such as hope, faith, and the ability to give and receive love, provide input into your psychological energy checking account. By maximizing these activities, you prepare to cope well with the stressors in your life just as having a large bank account helps you face a heavy financial burden.

Because stress is a complex phenomenon, it takes a multifaceted response to produce a high level of vital force to enable you to cope adequately with your stressors.

In the 1930s, Hans Selye became known as the father of stress research. Because of his pioneering work, we have realized that stress provokes a number of subtle chemical changes in the brain, which profoundly affect health. For example, stress produces deleterious effects on the immune system. The current data shows that the body's production of its own cancer-fighting cells, including what we call the natural killer cells (T-lymphocytes and macrophages) are inhibited by chronic stress.

Selye showed the three-step sequence of reaction to stress:

1. *The alarm reaction.* Often called the fight-or-flight syndrome, this instinctive physical change occurs when a threatening situation first confronts you, and your systems activate. Your voluntary muscles bulge, ready for action. At the same time, your heart rate and blood output increase, and the blood pressure is elevated. Blood sugar goes up and new stores are mobilized from the liver and muscles. Sensory perception increases. Your mouth becomes dry and perspiration increases. The spleen squeezes more blood cells into circulation and blood fats increase. Adrenal glands produce adrenaline that mobilizes your system into a state of emergency. This is a state of total alertness.

2. *Your system adjusts.* You adapt or resist. You're still on alert, but you take more time to make choices. You consider how to eliminate, modify, or avoid the stress. Your immune system adjusts to handle the situation. This may go on for days, even months. During this stage, most stress-related diseases develop. The problem occurs with individuals who continue to remain stressed, thus keeping their adrenaline system continually aroused. Your body wasn't made to live in a continuing state of arousal—it needs time to rest and recover from stimulation.

3. *Over a period of time, your system self-exhausts.* You use up your reserves, and you feel fatigued, disoriented, detached, or depressed. You may develop psychosomatic symptoms, such as headaches, backaches, muscle twitching, rashes, or wheezing. Sometimes you name this energy-deficient syndrome *burnout.*

Or you may go the other way and move into overadaptation. Instead of burnout, you conserve rather than exhaust your energy. You feel bored, cynical, unappreciated, depressed, disgusted, and may have serious self-doubts.

Long-term overstimulation causes such damaging effects as increased blood cholesterol and a decreased ability to remove the cholesterol from your blood. It encourages your blood platelets to stick together and elevates your blood pressure. All of these are causative factors for heart disease.

Modern research has shown that stress is an important causative element in coronary artery disease, hypertension, and stroke—the major causes of death in the Western world. Autoimmune diseases such as rheumatoid arthritis, lupus erythematosus, and myasthenia gravis also stem from stress.

When your brain is under negative stress, it manufactures an excess of a hormone called ACTH, which inhibits your body's production of white blood cells. These cells are vital in fighting off disease. Cancer as well as strokes and heart attacks are diseases of a weakened immune system. When your body becomes deficient in essential nutrients, you are less able to resist stressors. If these stressors stay with you for prolonged periods, such as weeks or even years, your body can't convert cholesterol into needed hormones, and you end up with exhaustion or some physical ailment. These physical breakdowns are your body's way of saying, "Enough! Treat me right and I'll treat you right." Too often, you probably don't listen.

> Stress begins in the mind but ends in the body.

STRESS AND TYPE A'S

In his 1974 book, *Type A Behavior and Your Heart,* Meyer Friedman introduced a new term to our vocabulary—*the Type A personality.* Although some critics say he oversimplified the research, his work still offers relevant information. He delineated the Type A as aggressive, high achievers, who are time and numbers oriented. They usually live with strained relationships.

Friedman contended that stress level, more than the other major risk factors (high fat, hypertension, lack of exercise, smoking) determines coronary artery disease in Type A people.

Type A individuals have two main hallmarks. First, they have the tendency to try to accomplish too many things in too little time. Second, they have a "free-floating" hostility. Trivial things irritate them, and they struggle against time as well as against other people. Type A traits develop in those who did not feel loved as children and who compensate as adults by proving their self-worth through what they do. Friedman suggested they have chronic, built-in distress.

One major factor of the Live-Longer Lifestyle studies, for those who want to live longer and healthier, is the control of stress. You need time for emotional growth, time to relax and enjoy your world.

LEARNING TO COPE

If you want to cope effectively with daily, ongoing stress, here are some suggestions.

1. *Exercise.* All parts of your body—the heart, kidneys, and intestines—become victims of chronic and excessive stress. An excellent way to deal with stress is to maintain a regular exercise program. It changes your hormonal system by increasing endorphins.

   In the middle of busy days, you might try deep-breathing exercises, or lift your shoulders toward your ears and drop them. As simple as these exercises are, they provide added energy and lessen your physical tension. You might enjoy playing tennis or golf. The form of exercise isn't as important as the fact that you *enjoy* the activity, because enjoyment contributes to building up your energy level.

2. *Eat right.* Following a good nutritional program allows you to store up the nutrients for energy in responding adequately to the fight-or-flight syndrome. Using some vitamin supplements during times of stress may also be a good idea to help you face these situations.

3. *Relax.* One way to restore your energy level is to rest. (You *can* cut back your fast-paced activities.) Some people meditate to relax. A technique practiced by many is Relaxation Response, developed by Dr. Herbert Benson of Harvard. He demonstrated that meditation sets off a built-in mechanism—the opposite of the fight-or-flight response. He suggested that stressed-out people learn to meditate for 10 to 20 minutes once or twice a day. Meditation produces a lasting reduction in blood pressure and other stress-related symptoms—natural antidotes to tension.

You can learn relaxation techniques quite easily. Get into a comfortable position, close your eyes, and concentrate on a single word, sound, or phrase. You could use the word *God* or *peace,* or concentrate on hearing ocean waves or the sound of running water. The idea is to be "passively unaware" of the outside world.

4. *Think right.* Your attitude is an important factor in keeping you at a high energy level. Taking a long-term outlook and seeing how your current challenge fits into the overall scheme of things can reduce the impact of stress. Maintaining a positive, optimistic attitude decreases the effects of stress and increases the immune system's response of producing killer T-cells.

One important way to boost your energy level is to exercise control over how you react. You need to learn to maintain a pace of life where your attitude controls the circumstances—they don't control you.

You can see this at work in part of a message Jesus gave his followers: "If someone strikes you on the right cheek, turn to him the other also. And if someone wants to sue you and take your tunic, let him have your cloak as well" (Matt. 5:39–40 NIV). He also referred to the practice that Romans could force Jews to carry the Romans' baggage for a mile. Jesus said, "Don't do it for a mile, but do it for two miles" (see Matt. 5:41).

By extending the distance, the oppressed had the freedom of making choices in situations that seemed to offer no choices. Those who chose to double the required distance were in charge of their decision and didn't take up the burden as a forced duty or feel subjugated.

Remember this principle as an excellent way to reduce stress: How you react to bad situations is your choice. By making the choice yourself, you build your energy level.

5. *Get support.* You need friends with good listening abilities, especially when you are challenged by stress. Not having friends, not

being involved in service organizations, or not belonging to church groups, can seriously affect your health.

Become a support person yourself. When you can make a contribution to a cause, or serve those who are more needy than yourself, it also builds your energy level.

6. *Think spiritually.* Modern science is beginning to realize the benefits of spirituality. Think about this fact: You have a Partner with whom you can share your burdens—Someone who freely provides advice and guidance. God is interested in your personal well-being.

Forgiving and not holding grudges can release you from stress. Jesus told us to love our neighbors as ourselves (Matt. 22:39). Love also implies forgiving. Jesus said to forgive seventy times seven, that is, indefinitely. (See Matt. 18:21–22.)

Love makes a powerful difference in our lives because it takes the focus off us (and our survival) and puts it on others. Many are able to face their stressors with a sparkle in their eyes and a smile on their faces. Using all of these factors can provide you with an energy level sufficient to cope well with stress.

This is borne out in the results of a survey of unemployed workers in the Detroit area by Louis Ferman of the University of Michigan. He referred to one man who defied the statistics and prognosis for high stress. That man had a rough employment history. In 1962, he lost his job when the Studebaker corporation went out of business. A decade later a truck manufacturer folded, and he lost his job again. In the 1980s, when Chrysler went through cutbacks, the man again lost his job.

"By all accounts, he should have been a basket case," Ferman said, "yet he was one of the best-adjusted fellows I've run into."

When asked his secret, the man said, "I've got a loving wife, and I go to church every Sunday."

Consider the stress that unnamed man must have gone

through during a thirty-year period. Yet he had positive forces to help him dispel the stress that might have torn another man apart.

Why focus on that Detroit man? Two reasons. First, because he's the exception. Second, because he had (perhaps unknowingly) learned how to overcome the stresses life had thrown at him.

GETTING PRACTICAL

You probably can't totally eliminate the powerful negative stresses in your life. But you can learn to win by overcoming their effects. Here are things you can do as you commit yourself to win over stress in life.

1. Identify the stress areas of your life. It may help you to list the things that irritate or worry you most. These might include marital problems, feelings of isolation, financial difficulties, too many commitments, work demands, problems with the family or children, lack of career direction, or lack of purpose in life.

2. Prioritize your tasks. Learn to prioritize by asking yourself if you really need to do certain tasks. Can you delegate them or turn them down? Can you do them at a later time? Are you doing them even though you don't want to or don't really need to?

   Rank your list with letters: A are the must-do tasks, B are the important tasks, C are things you would like to do, and D are those you will do if you have extra time and energy. Do the A tasks first. Finishing tasks brings satisfaction and a sense of accomplishment. Remind yourself that overloading leads you down the path to burnout.

3. Learn to adjust to stressors you can't avoid. You may need to adjust to conditions beyond your control. It can be as simple as saying to yourself, "If I want to work here, this is what I have to accept." You may need to learn to change your attitude toward those who provoke stress by accepting them as they are.

The Serenity Prayer used by Alcoholics Anonymous concludes with the words, "Give me the grace to accept those things I cannot change." Sometimes telling yourself, "This is part of life," may be enough to help you begin to accept this fact.

Dealing with stress means learning what is within your power to change and what isn't. You can only control yourself—you decide your actions.

4. Eliminate or modify stressful situations as much as possible. Avoid social situations where you feel stressed. Give up activities that increase the tension in your life, even though they may not be stress factors in themselves.

5. Learn to accept your limitations. Don't take on more than you can handle. Learn to say no to requests that overwhelm you and be realistic about what you can do.

6. Work off your tensions through exercise. Sometimes simply a change of pace will help.

7. Get physical. We say this a number of times in the book simply because it's so basic, and it's a factor that many resist. If you're feeling stressed, start with a healthy lifestyle. When your body is in good shape, you are better prepared for stress, and you can cope with life's pressures much more easily.

8. Relax. Remind yourself that not every situation is a life-or-death choice. One man in a high-pressure profession calms himself when he feels stress building by repeating, "This is only a job; it's not my entire life." He used to look at every aspect of his job as if it meant the end of his world if he didn't complete it fast and efficiently.

Now he works a little slower but doesn't feel exhausted at the end of the day.

9. Don't work at your job on your days off. (Don't let yourself get involved in mental-stress situations either.) Such occasions may arise, but ordinarily the habit of going back to the job when you need to rest isn't the best way to meet stress.

10. Learn to talk things out with those you trust. At times, you will find yourself in situations that get you down. Often just talking with a sympathetic person may be enough to release the tension. That person may be able to see your problem from a different angle and offer valuable insight.

11. Establish a support network. Our research shows that the spiritual and emotional support of the church rates high on the list of people who live healthier and longer lives. They've learned the value of discussing and sharing their problems. Someone once said that "support is the functional opposite of stress."

    A survey of nearly seven thousand residents in Alameda County, California, found that those with few such relationships had a death rate four times the rate of those who had many good, social relationships. Lonely, isolated people die sooner.

Perhaps you're awakening to the fact that even if you "have it all" in life—possessions, income, and achievement—it's still not enough. Fulfillment and a life of lower stress come when you are in harmonious relationship with other people, and even more, when you are in right relationship with the God who created you.

Health means success in living. Mental, physical, and spiritual health are assumed when you adjust well to life. Inner happiness depends not on external circumstances but on how you view yourself.

Positive attitudes and emotions help to produce positive chemical changes in your body that develop "happy hormones," endorphins— your body's natural opiates that give you a sense of well-being.

The most common factor in modern living is an unrealistic appraisal of what you deserve. The difference between what you think you deserve and what you actually receive causes stress. Just understanding this fact explains why gratitude is a powerful defense against stress-related illness.

Because I have chosen the healthier lifestyle,
I choose healthy ways to cope with stress.

A TIME TO REBUILD

THE LIGHTS went out and a quietness descended. Only the soft chirping of cicadas in the deep night broke the silence. As the day guard relaxed, the defense crew slowly began its nightly tasks, careful not to awaken the guard. Soundlessly, a central control system ordered workers to their stations. They brought in supplies and medicines and quietly repaired the ravages of the day's battles. All workers operated skillfully, efficiently, and without interruption. They had to finish within eight hours.

• • •

Exactly eight hours later, when the clanging of the alarm clock aroused the day guard, the others had finished their assigned tasks. For them, it had been a good night. The guard, now alert, was ready to fight for another day; they would return once again at nightfall to heal the day's wounds.

You have just read about sleep. You are the day guard. While you're awake, you use your energies as you move through the activities of your day. You're probably unaware that you're also causing wear in certain parts of your body. But once you fall asleep, your "defense crew" repairs the wounds, heals the sore places, and prepares you for the next day.

If you rested well—and long enough—last night, your night workers finished their work. They made you ready to start the day with vigor and alertness.

All of this because you had a good night's sleep.

The principle I want you to get is this: *You need to sleep well to stay well.*

Millions of Americans either don't understand that, or they consciously violate it in their sleep-deprived lives. Estimates say that as many as 30 percent of fatal automobile accidents happen when drivers fall asleep at the wheel. Research also suggests that at least one American in every twenty has caused an accident by nodding off while driving. Most such accidents occur between midnight and 6:00 A.M. The root of the problem is not the long drives, the late hours, the boredom of expressways, or the lack of light but an unwillingness to admit the need for sleep because of the hyperactive American lifestyle.

One expert said that *every day* 100 million sleep-deprived Americans are driving cars and trucks, operating hazardous machinery, administering medical care, monitoring nuclear power plants, and even piloting commercial jets.

Sleep deprivation affects 30 to 50 percent of the population, and a large number of people go without sufficient sleep on a fairly regular basis.

Americans are shaving hours off their sleep to work longer, spend more time with their family, do household chores, play golf, or chat on the Internet. Teens are staying up late to work, study, and socialize and then getting up early the next day for school.

Sleep simply isn't a high priority. Worse, many people have been sleepy for so long, they don't know what it's like to feel wide awake. Chances are that every one of those sleep-deprived people is less than fully alert and is performing below par. Many are so sleepy that they are likely to nod off while reading, listening to a lecture, driving on a monotonous road, or flying an aircraft. The FAA has documented a number of cases in which, although they didn't fall asleep, pilots' ability to be alert to crucial details became impaired.

Many blame sleep deprivation on our twenty-four-hour society, where electric lights, twenty-four-hour businesses, TV sets, and electronic highways encourage us to put off going to sleep. People must depend on alarm clocks to get going in the mornings. Many sleep-deprived people even brag about their less-than-adequate sleep.

Try this sometime. Get into a conversation with friends and start talking about sleep. "I only need five hours of sleep," one person will say quickly. Others will probably either try to beat that number or explain how they have learned to function with less sleep. In some circles, it's considered laziness to admit to needing eight hours of sleep each night.

The simple fact:

If you want good health, you can't do without adequate sleep and rest.

Sleep and rest are part of God's plan for human life—for your life. It's the daily time for your body to rebuild and to recover from the stresses of the hours you're awake. Rest is an important part of the rhythm of life.

It might interest you to know that in the 1800s, people averaged *nine and a half hours* of sleep each night. A century later the figure had dropped to eight hours. One study followed the rapidity of the trend toward sleep deprivation. It said that by the early 1980s, Americans averaged only seven and a half hours sleep. In the 1990s, the average had dropped to a little less than seven hours.

By contrast, when we did a random sample survey among those who embrace the Live-Longer Lifestyle, most averaged eight hours of sleep each night—another reason for their longevity and better health.

This lack of adequate rest concerns those of us who care about America's health. You may have cut down on sleep to get more things done. But do you really accomplish more? You can't fool your body. You—like every other human being in the world—have an individual, biological need for a certain amount of sleep. A few people can get by on six hours; others need as many as nine.

While you can't fool your body, you can cheat it—for a time. It's like borrowing from the bank—one day you have to pay it back. You can live with lesser amounts of sleep and vast amounts of caffeine or other stimulants to keep you going. One day, however, your body will rebel through physical sickness, an accident, or traumatic problems. You can't continue to abuse your body (and sleep deprivation is abuse!) and not expect to have to account for it later.

Experts haven't agreed on how we must pay off "sleep debts" or what the consequences of long-term sleep deficits are. Yet as one person pointed out, "As people continue to cut back on sleep, they tread a narrower and narrower path. Some are walking on a thin tightrope."

The Live-Longer Lifestyle studies agree: If you want to maximize your health and longevity, you must get the amount of sleep your body needs.

Sleeping is not a waste of time. Think of what happens when you sleep. Your nonworking period is time for your body and mind to restore energy and re-create health.

Think about how your heart works. For every heart contraction (systole), you have a brief rest period (diastole). If your heart is healthy, it contracts in about 1/10 of a second. The remainder of that second it *rests*. During the resting period, oxygen and nutrients nourish the heart and enable it to continue at peak efficiency.

Your kidneys also function on this work-rest principle. The filters of the kidneys operate in three shifts: one-third of the cycle in action, one-third in rest, and one-third in preparation for action. All through your body you can find this work-rest cycle. Each cell has a function to perform. Not getting enough rest results in the depletion of the working force of each cell.

Think about the last time you did strenuous labor or exercised for an extended period. When you stopped (maybe from exhaustion), you had to rest, didn't you? Once you rested, you could begin again.

Your body has that built-in rhythm. You can cooperate with it or fight it. If you listen to the rhythm of your body, you are in tune with yourself.

Are you one of those who tries to move to a fast march (4/4 time), when your body requests a slow waltz (3/4 time)? If so, you probably get ahead of the music, out of sync—and eventually, your health will suffer. That is, you get sick. Your body simply says, "I've had enough. I'm going to force you to rest—now."

Isn't it interesting that when the so-called flu season comes along, doctors prescribe rest as a key ingredient to recovery? Maybe this should tell us something important.

WHAT HAPPENS WHEN YOU SLEEP

When you're asleep, your senses temporarily shut down. They still function, but your brain doesn't encode them. In deep sleep, you aren't conscious of anything that your memory records.

When you're awake, your body concentrates on action and motion. Hormones, such as epinephrine and glycogen, use up your body's proteins. You have no extra energy to repair or replace worn-out parts. During the hours of sleep, your body does the repair work. The hormonal balance shifts to an anabolic or building mode. Insulin, testosterone, and other building hormones make new proteins for your body.

Sleep has more value than just passing time when you're too tired to work. It's when you prepare for another day. Your body makes muscle tissue, blood components, and even builds bones during those hours of repose.

Sleep clinics report that we move back and forth between light sleep and deep sleep four or five times in an eight-hour period. Today, the common classification is to refer to REM (rapid eye movement) or synchronized sleep and NREM (no rapid eye movement) or desynchronized sleep.

When you enter REM sleep, your muscles relax, you have little activity except for eye movement, and your dreams seem more vivid. If you awaken during this period, you can probably recall your dream.

If you're getting proper amounts and quality of sleep, REM makes up 20 to 25 percent of your total sleep.

If your body doesn't get enough REM sleep one night, it tries to make up for it the next. You then have a "rebound" in which you spend more than the usual amount of time in REM sleep.

In laboratory settings, researchers have shown that when they awaken subjects whenever they are having rapid eye movement, they will awaken them approximately five times the first night. Because of this disruption, during the following night, the researchers will have to awaken the subjects more frequently because they have more REM periods. It's as if their bodies say, "I didn't get enough last night, so I'm making it up tonight."

WHEN IS ENOUGH ENOUGH?

No one knows exactly how much sleep anyone needs. You have a unique body rhythm. You may be an early riser and do your most productive work in the morning hours. If so, you shouldn't agree to take on a project that requires intense concentration at night. Or you may be the type who just can't get your peak feeling until the middle of the morning or even in the late afternoon.

Regardless of whether you peak early in the day or late at night, you need sleep. If you deprive yourself, you interfere with your body's work-and-rest function. This interference affects your efficiency *and eventually your health*. Studies have shown that if people go without sleep for prolonged periods of time, they begin to hallucinate and take on paranoiac behavior. (Some people have a highly efficient sleep system. For instance, they may "catnap" once, twice, or even three times in twenty-four hours and not seem to need as much sleep as others. Apparently, Thomas Edison needed less than four hours of sleep. But Edison was an exception.)

The amount of sleep you need for good health is something you have to figure out for yourself—and it's not difficult. The amount not only differs with each individual, but we also believe age has something to do with it. Newborns sleep up to twenty hours a day. Young children need up to twelve hours of sleep. By age forty, most of us need seven or eight hours. After age forty, the need increases slightly for the next thirty years. After that, the amount of sleep needed tends to decline again.

These increases and decreases relate to brain metabolism. The more active your brain, the more sleep you need. Newborns have almost twice the brain activity of young children, so they require twice as much sleep. If you need nine hours of sleep, it may be because you use so much of your brain while you're awake that you need to put it into the shop for more extensive maintenance.

In the 1973 Alameda County study of approximately seven thousand men and women ages thirty to seventy, researchers learned that those who regularly slept seven to eight hours a night had the lowest death rates. Those who slept more than eight hours or less than seven had significantly higher death rates.

ARE YOU GETTING ENOUGH SLEEP?

Consider the following information to see if you're getting enough sleep.

- If you're not getting enough sleep, you probably nod off whenever you're not active—sitting in church, watching TV, even driving your car. It's not that such activities induce sleep, but quiet activities bring out the need to rest.

- If you need an alarm to wake up, you're probably sleep deprived. If you are providing for your biological sleep need, your brain awakens on its own.

- If you sleep longer on your days off, it probably means you're not getting enough sleep on the other nights.

HOW MUCH SLEEP DO *YOU* NEED?

If you're ready to find out exactly how much sleep you need, here is an easy way to do it. Say you're averaging six hours of sleep a night. Set aside a week, such as vacation time, where you can spend up to nine hours in bed. If you sleep eight or nine hours the first night or two, you may be repaying your sleep debt. After the second or third night, do you continue to need nine hours? Have you dropped back to seven? If you continue to awaken after eight hours, that's your body's wise way of saying, "Hey, this is what I need."

Listen to your body's wisdom. If you really can't sleep more than seven hours and you wake up on your own, you're probably getting enough sleep.

In Western cultures, a typical pattern is to squeeze by on five hours of sleep and "make it up" on the weekends by sleeping ten to twelve hours. Experts are divided on whether you can repay your sleep debt that way; however, they agree that you probably won't have any permanent bad effects from this. Studies indicate, however, that you only make up about 75 percent of your lost sleep. For example, if you go without sleep for two days and then sleep the second night, probably you won't sleep sixteen hours, but will tend to awaken after twelve.

This much researchers agree on: The best sleep comes from uninterrupted periods of six or seven hours. Thirty-minute naps help to relax you and break down the stress, but not everyone is a napper. John F. Kennedy and Sir Winston Churchill were legendary nappers. Both claimed to feel fully refreshed after a half-hour's sleep in the middle of the day.

GETTING THE MOST OUT OF YOUR SLEEP

One way to ensure that you get a good night's rest is to *not* eat before going to bed. Popular wisdom says that you need a snack before you turn in for the night. Research indicates that you get the best sleep if you have a period of at least four hours between the last ingestion of food and sleep.

If you go to bed on a full stomach, you may awaken tired, even if you sleep sufficient hours. A full stomach can interfere with your rest because your body is too busy finishing up the digestive work to rest. Common sense says that you'll sleep better and awaken more refreshed if you go to sleep on an empty stomach.

Note that a heavy meal before bedtime also adds extra stress on your heart. It increases the number of fat particles in the circulating blood, which can set you up for a heart attack while you sleep. This explains why 52 percent of heart attacks occur when people are sleeping or resting.

Insomnia is the most common of all sleep problems, and it's difficult to treat. It consists of difficulty either in falling asleep or in staying asleep. Emotional disturbances, such as depression and anxiety, have caused all of us periods of insomnia. Do you sometimes find you can't sleep because you anticipate an exciting event, such as the start of a new job? entering college? getting married? leaving for vacation? worrying about downsizing at work? Researchers estimate that about 50 percent of Americans occasionally have insomnia.

Occasional insomnia need not concern you. But if you are persistently unable to sleep, you may need help. Taking drugs isn't a cure; they only treat symptoms and don't get to the cause. While some tranquilizers offer periods of sleep without interfering with REM sleep, they usually work only for short periods of time. And many sleep aids inhibit REM sleep, leaving you feeling unrested.

We now know that certain drugs can cause insomnia. Caffeine is probably the most widely used drug that affects sleep.

If you have insomnia, we suggest that you get a medical checkup. If your physician can find no physical cause, you may wish to speak to a counselor or therapist. Start by asking yourself: What's eating away at me that won't allow me to relax?

GETTING PRACTICAL

1. Establish a regular, daily sleep schedule. Go to bed at the same time and get up at the same time, including *weekends*. Even if you don't feel sleepy at your regular bedtime at first, stay in your routine for at least one month.

2. Avoid late-night snacks. Get into a regular eating schedule. It's best if you don't eat for at least four hours before you go to sleep. Avoid snacking or drinking anything with caffeine.

3. Avoid alcohol; it suppresses essential REM sleep.

4. Try to sleep in a quiet room.

5. Relax your body before you try to sleep. Drink a cup of warm, herbal tea. Take a lukewarm bath or shower. A whirlpool is excellent.

6. Sleep in a well-ventilated room. Avoid drafts, but make sure you have indirect air flow through open windows or ceiling fans.

7. Develop a regular exercise program, especially if you have a sedentary job or you have a lot of pressure or emotional fatigue.

8. End your day with quietness. Avoid any heavy physical workout or mental high near the end of the day. Read or listen to music—whatever you find relaxing.

9. Count your blessings. Lie quietly and see how many things you can think of for which you're thankful. Allow these quiet thoughts to relax you.

10. If you don't fall asleep immediately, don't be concerned. You can teach your body to relax. If you rest quietly for six or seven hours, you will get enough restorative rest to handle the next day. Don't lie in bed and worry about not being able to sleep.

  You will likely get sleep you're not aware of. Consistently, sleep studies show that subjects get more sleep than they realize.

Some have found that when they can't sleep, they turn to music or reading. They absorb themselves in this activity, and it soon induces sleep.

11. Aim for balance in your schedule. It's one more way to take control over your health. Rest is essential for your body to rebuild and repair worn parts and develop the energy to retain control of your health. Developing the personal power and desire to be in charge is one of the benefits of resting and relaxing.

Because I want to live longer and healthier,
I get the sleep I need each night.

HOW TO RELAX

If you're one of those individuals who simply doesn't know how to relax, this is for you. You *can* learn simple, health-extending ways to let go of tension.

Method 1

Lie comfortably on your back. Do this exercise to a slow count of eight:

1. Concentrate on your entire right leg as you silently say "one" slowly. Visualize your entire leg relaxing, beginning at the toes and moving upward. Think of your entire body as slowly descending into calm.

2. Concentrate on your left leg as you say "two" silently and slowly. Again, visualize your entire leg relaxing from the toes upward and think of your entire body as slowly descending into calm.

3. At "three," do the same with your right arm, relaxing from the fingertips upward.

4. At "four," repeat with your left arm.

5. On the count of "five," visualize all the muscles of your back relaxing.

6. At "six," include your waist to your thighs.

7. When you say "seven," concentrate on your upper body.

8. Finally, as you say "eight," visualize letting go of the tension in your head. Make sure your jaws are relaxed. Imagine a calmness flowing inside your skull.

If you aren't fully relaxed go through the exercise again.

Method 2

Lie comfortably on your back. Do this exercise to a slow count of seven:

1. Clench your fists. Be aware of the tension all the way to your shoulders.

2. Open your hands. Think about the relaxation in your arms.

3. Bend your toes and feet downward. Be aware of the tension throughout your legs.

4. Release and feel the tension drain away from your legs.

5. Close your eyes tightly and press your lips together. Bite down hard.

6. Relax your eyes, lips, and jaw.

7. Take a deep breath and relax your whole body. Feel yourself melt into whatever you're lying on.

If you aren't fully relaxed go through the exercise again.

MOBILIZING DEFENSES

INVADERS STEALTHILY surround the sacred temple. Silently, they take up their offensive positions and prepare to attack.

• • •

They don't realize they will lose the upcoming battle. The *one* significant factor in their impending loss is a highly trained team of lymphocyte paratroopers called NK-cells, standing watch for the first sign of invasion. Always ready to mobilize their forces and fight off all invaders, they patrol the sacred temple. Although they can't stop the invasions, they can throw off any attacks.

As you visualize this situation, picture yourself as that sacred temple. Every day, enemies attempt to destroy your temple. The battles are waged around you and inside you. You can win each skirmish only if your natural killer cells stay vigilant. Anything that weakens your energy, health, alertness, and perception gives the invaders an advantage.

Your enemies—bacteria, viruses, cancer cells, fungi—assault your body through any opening—your mouth, eyes, nose, an open sore, or even skin pores. Pollutants, chemicals, and stress continually barrage your body.

How will you handle the next onslaught? Will you lose the battle this winter to a flu bug? Get felled by a nasty cold? Let a bronchial infection knock you out of action for a week? Or will you take charge and fight?

Whether you know it or not, you have power over the organisms and environmental poisons that invade your body. You have everything you need to win and keep on winning indefinitely. Colds and flu bugs are everywhere, but you don't have to succumb. Set your elite team free to do its job, and let it ward off the encroaching attack.

Do you assume you'll have to put up with your yearly bout with the flu? "It's the curse of modern life," one man said.

It doesn't have to be.

The best way to prove this point is to look at adherents of the Live-Longer Lifestyle. Ask them how many days of sickness they have experienced during the past year. The past ten or twenty years? Ask them about their bouts with bronchitis or a urinary infection. Most of them probably can't remember because it's been too many years.

Jan has had only a couple of colds since 1980.

Cec used to come down with a nasty cold every January—a week or so after the hectic holiday season. Then he learned to take care of himself. He has not had one cold since 1985.

Thousands of people have learned how to live a healthier lifestyle that fights off colds and infections. That they live longer is simply a bonus; they're more interested in enjoying and preserving the lifestyle they have now. You can enjoy the same freedom from sickness.

It's not easy, but you can do it.

You can live healthier as you live longer, but it will take discipline and sensible care.

Think about this: Every day you are exposed to thousands of germs. Many of them are part of your daily life—already present and waiting to take advantage when your defenses are run down. In the microscopic world, the rule is kill or be killed. Your immune systems fight for you every day of your life.

Your superb surveillance-and-defense system is designed to protect you from disease, whether it's sinus infection or cancer. Your complex defense system consists of various components, such as the thymus gland, bone marrow, spleen, and lymph system. All parts of your immune system combine to create a fighting force of intricate complexity that takes on tumors, bacteria, and viruses, as well as an assortment of yeasts, fungi, and parasites.

The enemy troops are invisible without the magnification of a microscope. When they successfully breach your lines of defense, their collective presence is called an *infection*.

Infections have names, such as tuberculosis, leprosy, malaria, influenza, or the common cold. Some have exotic names: the Hong Kong flu, Ebola virus, bubonic plague, or AIDS.

YOUR IMMUNE SYSTEM

How does your immune system's defense work against the powerful forces of infection? To begin with, your immune cells are born in the bone marrow. Every day, your bone marrow pours out millions of new red and white blood cells. The red cells carry oxygen, and the white cells act as your guard against disease.

Say you get a small cut on your finger. Immediately you come under attack by germs that enter the cut on your finger and rapidly multiply. They actually multiply exponentially. (That means two become four and four become sixteen.) They secrete their toxins and, if your body allows them to carry on their reproductive cycles, soon turn into a powerful invading force.

Your white corpuscles, however, are ready for such an invasion. A silent chemical alarm goes off when you cut your finger. The blood in the immediate area of the wound starts to get sticky. Blood cells hop up on the capillary vessel walls and slow the blood down. Blood cells keep arriving and make the area slightly swollen and tender. This is called an *inflammatory response*.

Within moments of cutting yourself, your white blood cells crawl through the capillary walls. They leave the blood vessels and head for the site of the invasion where the battle rages. The first troops surround the invading germs and fight. Your white troops that die in battle become *pus*. The surviving troops continue to clean up the area until you have defeated the invaders.

Most of your immune cells are nonspecific fighters, like foot soldiers, who will go after anything that threatens you. You also have an elite killer force called lymphocytes, the elite combat officers, white blood cells that attack specific targets. You have four main categories of lymphocytes: T-cells, B-cells, NK-cells, and macrophages. They all come from the bone marrow. The B-cells go immediately to your lymph nodes, tonsils, spleen, and certain tissues in your gut where they fight for your health. Those that will become T-cells go to the thymus, a two-lobed gland in the upper portion of the chest at the base of the neck. When they later emerge from the thymus, they function as T-cells and direct the NK-cells (natural killer cells).

Macrophages are the national guard and are stationed in various parts of your body. Some researchers say the reason macrophages have decreased in effectiveness in modern America is because of a combination of lifestyle changes, nutritional deficiency, and especially the overuse of antibiotics.

T-cells identify the invader, obtain a picture or sample of the invader, and send a message either to the NK-cells to kill the invaders or to the B-cells to produce antibodies to immobilize or destroy the enemy. NK-cells work best because they're equipped for hand-to-hand combat. B-cells hurl chemical missiles. That is, NK-cells bump up against the enemy to fight, while the B-cells kill from a distance. If this nonspecific kill effect goes awry and fights against the body instead of the invaders, the result is called an autoimmune disease. These include diabetes, asthma, arthritis, and colitis.

Your healthy troops fight against external enemies, *germs*. This term refers to microorganisms, viruses, bacteria, and other life forms we don't know about. (Yet these germs alone are not the cause of the cold you had last fall or the flu you had during the winter.)

Viruses are responsible for everything from influenza and hepatitis to polio, rabies, some forms of cancer, and AIDS.

Bacteria cause such life-threatening diseases as tetanus, tuberculosis, syphilis, and toxic shock. They also contaminate your food and cause food poisoning, including the deadly botulism.

Did you know this?

Not all the bacteria in your body are bad. Some produce enzymes that break down food molecules so you can assimilate them. Other bacteria produce pigment. Still others are active in essential chemical processes.

Germs are inside and around you all the time. They don't just show up when the weather turns bad or when you get your feet wet. In a world teeming with microscopic activity, you probably carry about 100 trillion bacteria internally or externally all the time. You are constantly exposed to potential disease producers. The good news is that if you are average, you are symptom-free most of the time. Given the concentration of germs in your immediate surroundings, if they were the only cause of disease, you would constantly be ill with something.

Have you ever noticed that the flu bug goes through an entire office or workplace in a period of about a month? Have you also noticed that a few workers never come down with that forty-eight-hour virus? Or you may have observed one or two family members who seem immune to disease. Are those people just lucky? In any epidemic, a certain number of caregivers have no protection, yet they don't succumb. The Ebola virus that hit Africa in 1995 took hundreds of lives. Yet not everyone who came in contact with the disease caught it.

There is a reason.

When your body is healthy—meaning more than just symptom-free—disease-producing bacteria can't penetrate your defenses.

Bad germs can't affect health unless they can penetrate cells. They can't penetrate your cells unless your body's vitality and resistance are reduced. Resistance reducers include accidents, poor diet, excessive fatigue, or high levels of stress. Short-term, high-intensity events (i.e., accidents) or the long-term abuse of a destructive lifestyle disrupts the normal function of the body as a whole, as well as the cells that make it up.

All pathogenic germs (those harmful to the body) are scavengers. They don't attack healthy cells or tissue; they feed on damaged cells. If you keep yourself fit, you can peacefully coexist with your germs and stay healthy.

If they are strong and prepared, your NK-cells will fight. But if you ignore your immune system's basic needs, even your elite forces won't fight. When a major microbe attacks, your defense forces will be too tired to leave the barracks. You may end up in the doctor's office or the hospital.

You can take charge of your health by caring for your immune system. Do this by living a balanced life and giving your immune system the opportunity to be in optimal shape to defend you.

"Then why do so many people get sick?" you may ask.

There are two reasons. Either they don't live a balanced life, or they have what we call a variation in their immune protective systems—some people have exceptionally weak systems.

Your best protection is to make sure your cells stay healthy enough to keep your vitality at its peak. Lifestyle is the primary determinant of health—what you eat, how you treat your body, the quality of your rest, and your attitude. If you're angry, worried, hyperactive, or a complainer, you're a prime candidate for chronic disease and early death.

You have a physiological response every time any of your five senses is stimulated by food, activities, smells, visual impressions, memories, environment, or attitudes, such as anger or frustration. These responses affect your cells. Negative responses weaken your defenses. It's that simple—and yet amazingly complex. When you reduce the vitality of your cells, you affect your entire body and reduce your resistance to disease.

Symptoms of pain, discomfort, fever, nausea, or other signs of disease develop according to the type of trauma suffered and your individual response. If you scrape your knee in a fall, your symptoms appear immediately. Other ailments, such as heart disease, take longer to show up.

When your symptoms get uncomfortable or interfere with your daily routine, you'll probably do something about them. You may consult a doctor who prescribes medication, or you may treat yourself with over-the-counter drugs. Although these drugs may relieve your symptoms, they likely won't cure the problem.

Antibiotics often chase bacteria away. Unfortunately, germs can also adapt to their environment. More and more bacteria are becoming resistant to drugs that once kept them in line. Another problem is that most antibiotics go after the helpful bacteria as vigorously as they go after the harmful ones. Drugs may kill bacteria, but unless the resistance of the hosts is improved, the same or another variety of invaders will strike again.

HOW YOUR BODY FIGHTS

When your resistance is low and the germs attack, you may develop such symptoms as a runny nose or watery eyes. Think of that as your body's attempt to maintain health. Its first defense is dilution—diluting substances your body doesn't need makes them less harmful. Although a cold makes you feel rotten, your sneezing and runny nose serve a purpose. Your body is getting rid of toxins that can threaten your survival. As long as you can develop a good cold, you know that your body can still fight.

The same is true of fevers. High temperatures kill off pathogenic bacteria that live best in the normal 98.6°F environment. Up to about 104°F, a fever burns off toxic materials and allows your body to resume its regular routine. The next time you get a fever, think of it as a health-restorer.

But even better, why allow yourself to get run down and put up with fevers and sneezing? They don't have to be part of your life.

Many people experience wonderful results in fighting colds with echinacea, a natural herb. They take one capsule every three to four hours for one or two days at the onset of a cold. Some notice the symptoms disappearing after the first two or three pills. Others add vitamin C or garlic capsules and speak of significant improvement. Many physicians recognize the effectiveness of echinacea and suggest its use in treating colds.

GETTING PRACTICAL

Here are suggestions for strengthening your immune system so that you win most battles.

1. Satisfy your vitamin and mineral needs. If you're not sure you're getting adequate nutrients, you may want to look into taking supplements. However, if you decide to use supplements, do so at a modest level.

   - *Vitamin A.* Get plenty of vitamin A, which helps to activate disease-fighting T-cells. This vitamin occurs in yellow, orange, and dark-green fruits and vegetables, such as squash, carrots, cantaloupe, spinach, broccoli, sweet potatoes, and apricots. Vitamin A is in leafy greens, such as spinach, kale, mustard greens, and collards. Beta carotene is a form of vitamin A that specializes in fighting invaders. You'll get all you need if you eat the yellow and orange foods.

   - *B vitamins.* Certain B vitamins also bolster your immunity, especially B_6. You'll get large amounts of B_6 in refried beans, wild rice, garbanzos, navy beans, and baked potatoes.

- *Vitamin C.* Don't overlook vitamin C; it stimulates the production of interferon, a chemical that "interferes" with the reproduction of viruses and stops them from spreading. Interferon also helps to destroy tumors. You'll find vitamin C in citrus fruits, broccoli, brussels sprouts, pea pods, and kohlrabi.

- *Vitamin E.* The antioxidant vitamin E plays a significant role in preventing age-related decline in your immune system. Filberts, almonds, garbanzos, most vegetable oils, and whole wheat are all excellent sources.

- *Iron.* Iron does more than build healthy blood; it also enables you to fight infections. This mineral makes hemoglobin, the protein that carries oxygen to your cells. (A healthy supply of oxygen destroys invading bacteria.) You'll probably get enough iron if you eat daily amounts of such foods as spinach, potatoes, broccoli, cashews, soybeans, and lima beans.

- *Zinc.* You need zinc for more than eighty functions of your body. It's crucial to many parts of the immune system. Zinc deficiency is common among the elderly and makes them susceptible to infections.

  When researchers put a group of elderly people on vitamin and mineral supplements for several months without any other dietary change, their immune systems reached a level of activity equal to that of twenty-year-olds. Almonds, cashews, peanuts, and pecans are excellent sources of zinc.

- *Calcium.* Calcium is the binding surface that allows the natural killer cells to attach to tumor cells and destroy them. You'll get a good supply in broccoli, almonds, collards, garbanzos, and navy beans.

- *Magnesium.* Found in nuts and whole grains, magnesium helps to prevent disease.

- *Selenium.* Selenium works with vitamin E to provide fuel to your antibodies. Brazil nuts and kohlrabi, as well as some cereals, are rich sources of selenium.

2. Wash your hands before meals and after using the bathroom. Your parents and teachers insisted that you practice good hygiene. Because germs on your hands tend to end up in your mouth, washing helps to prevent infections. A quick rinse with soap and water is generally enough.

3. Scrub all your fruits and vegetables clean, especially if you're going to eat them raw. Cut mold spots from firm vegetables such as cabbage and carrots. If mold appears on your fruits or soft vegetables such as tomatoes, cucumbers, and lettuce, discard them. Also throw away any moldy soft cheese, cottage cheese, cream, sour cream, yogurt, or individual cheese slices.

4. After preparing food, keep it hot or keep it cold. Don't let a hot dish cool on the counter before you put it in the refrigerator because that's when bacteria get in. Thaw frozen foods in the refrigerator.

5. Quit eating sweets. You probably won't like this, but it's one way to keep your immune system operating at peak efficiency. Candy, ice cream, and pastries are loaded with sugar that cripples your white blood cells and keeps them from destroying viruses and bacteria. The higher your sugar intake, the more it depresses your immune system.

   "You mean I have to give up all sweets?" you may be asking.

   The answer is no, but be moderate. When you sense a cold coming on, cut out sugar entirely. Instead, drink a lot of water, and you'll do your immune system a favor.

6. Get physical. Moderate exercise stimulates your body's natural killer cells' activities. They can slow tumor growth or help to make

one vanish. Ride a stationary bicycle. Develop a pleasant fitness activity, such as walking, to stimulate your production of endorphins. They help eradicate germs. Try a 20-minute walk during your lunch break.

7. Don't exercise to the point of exhaustion, such as running a marathon. Exhaustion depresses your killer cells' activities for up to 24 hours.

   Lee Berk, D.H.Sc. at Loma Linda University, in a study of marathon runners, discovered that the athletes' immune systems (specifically NK-cells) were depressed for 6 hours after competition—a good time for illness to strike.

8. Get involved in helping others. Make a decision to do something good for someone else at least once a week. It could be as easy as taking a bag of groceries to a needy family or paying someone's utility bill. Visit someone in a nursing home. Call a shut-in. Write a letter to encourage someone you know who's depressed. You could read for the blind, cook for the ill, pass on your good clothing, or send cards to those who are sick.

   "Studies of volunteers have shown that not only do they tend to live longer, but also they often feel better, sometimes reporting a sudden burst of endorphins similar to a 'runner's high' while helping others," says Dean Ornish.[1]

9. Improve your emotional outlook. The relatively new field of psychoneuroimmunology addresses the connections between your emotions, your brain, and your immune system. Negative emotions suppress your immune system, while positive emotions cause it to soar. This means that if you're hostile, afraid, or depressed, you're more likely to get sick. If you are optimistic, caring, and trusting, you're more likely to stay well.

   Research now links negative emotions to the suppression of the immune system. One study found a link between the depression of widowers after their wives' deaths and a drop in the ability of their lymphocytes to fight. Another report referred to a twenty-year study of electric company workers. It said that depressed employees were almost twice as likely to die of a deadly disease as those with a more positive emotional state.

All of the advice above is to stress that *you are responsible for your own life.* Feeling in control of what's happening in your life enhances your immune system.

10. Learn to manage stress. Use deep breathing exercises and practice relaxation techniques for 15 minutes a day. Take some time to relax and just think.

11. Rethink your goals in life. If you want to improve your lifestyle and live healthier, then make getting a good night's sleep on a regular basis one of your goals. A good night's sleep is one of the best ways to rebuild your immune system.

12. Develop an optimistic attitude. Don't take yourself too seriously.

13. Plan fun activities with your family or friends. Play games. Arrange activities that will help you laugh and enjoy your life. Get away to the mountains or the ocean to relax and enjoy companionship.

14. Cut out all substances that reduce the effectiveness of your defense system. You already know them: nicotine, alcohol, coffee and other caffeinated drinks, recreational drugs. Avoid high-risk behavior.

15. Drink six to eight glasses of water every day. Your cells need that much water to enhance your immune system.

16. Maintain your immunizations and have your doctor check your lymphocyte levels. Know what they are and try to keep them up.

---

*Because I want to live longer and healthier,
I maintain a healthy immune system—my marvelous
defense system.*

TAKE IT EASY!

CHAPTER 17

WHAT *REALLY* happened to Jim Fixx—the legendary runner of the 1980s?

• • •

He completed twenty marathons, averaged running 60 miles a week, and recorded that he ran a total of 37,000 miles. The news stunned runners around the world when Fixx died of a heart attack at age fifty-two after completing a mere 4-mile run. An autopsy revealed that his coronary arteries were almost blocked, and he had scar tissue from two previous heart attacks.

Many people accepted that he had died as the result of a genetic heart condition—which was true enough—but a decade passed before researchers understood the cause of his death.

We can sum up the major cause in a single word: *moderation*—or the lack of it—in the life of Jim Fixx. Those who knew him spoke of his terrible eating habits and lifestyle. Ultra-marathon runner Stan Cottrell said he and Fixx appeared together at a conference. Just before Fixx went in to speak, he "stuffed himself with four donuts and said, 'I didn't have time for breakfast.'"

That was typical of Fixx's eating habits. He depended on his intense running schedule to keep him fit. Unfortunately, he had it figured wrong. It was his lifestyle (including the lack of moderation), not just genetics, that killed him.

God gave us bodies that can tolerate almost anything—in small amounts. Moderation is one of the key health principles in taking care of ourselves. This principle reminds us that we can go too far—even with good things.

It's not easy to be moderate. It requires some amount of self-discipline. However, those who temper what they eat and drink have significantly fewer health problems. Moderation in food choices and activities profoundly affects energy level *and longevity*.

MODERATION IN EATING

Moderation means taking reasonable care in what and how much you eat. Let's think for a moment about the somewhat frequent practice of overeating. In addition to the feeling of lethargy and lack of energy often associated with overeating, you face the prospect of another, more long-term consequence: weight gain.

Another place to stress moderation is in fat intake. Although researchers had suspected that a low-fat diet was beneficial, it wasn't until 1935 that Dr. Clive McCay of Cornell University produced hard evidence to show its importance. He used the experimental evidence to extend the average maximum life span, postpone the onset of catastrophic disease and decrease the frequency of most or all of the aging diseases, maintain biomarkers at levels below chronological age, maintain sexual potency into advanced ages, and delay deterioration of the brain.

McCay demonstrated that rats on a calorically restrictive but healthy diet supplemented with vitamins and minerals lived much longer than normally fed rats. By 1,000 days, all the normally fed rats had died; most of the calorie-restricted ones were alive and active. Their growth rate and body size had been retarded by the severely restrictive regimen, but in other ways they seemed super healthy. If they were allowed a full diet at 1,000 days, they actually began to grow again. The females were sexually active and could reproduce far beyond the normal age. The males had higher testosterone levels than normally fed older males.

The maximum life spans of McCay's restricted rats reached 1,800 days—the equivalent of 150 to 180 human years. He couldn't, of course, replicate this with humans. The severe food restrictions kept the rats from reaching full body size, and they would affect humans the same way. The experiment, however, definitely proved that maximum life span can be greatly extended.

While some could argue that this research refers only to rats, scientists have replicated these experiments in a variety of species with short life spans. Naturally, it will take many years before they can demonstrate this in humans—if they ever do. However, as they examine the effects of human overeating, they point to the resulting diseases, such as diabetes, hypercholesterolemia, and hypertension, that shorten human life span.

McCay's pioneering work strongly suggests that aging isn't irretrievably fixed by some unyielding law of nature.

In recent years, a number of research centers have confirmed his data. For example, in 1967 researchers at UCLA applied his findings to human beings. The results indicated that in adulthood, the caloric restriction works best when implemented *slowly*. Imposing caloric restriction too rapidly actually seems to shorten the life span. *Crash diets and prolonged fasting probably shorten survival.* The body needs time to adapt to change—even to a more healthful lifestyle.

MODERATION IN EXERCISE

Let's look at another arena where moderation is important: exercise.

Dr. Kenneth Cooper, who invented the term *aerobics,* says that excessive exercise is dangerous, while a moderate program is helpful.

A marathon runner himself, he became disturbed that during the final weeks of training for a marathon, he frequently came down with a viral type of illness, such as a cold or the flu. At the very time he needed to concentrate intently on his training, sickness forced him into a few days of nonactivity. He believes his excessive training actually worked against his fitness.

Along the same lines, David C. Nieman, then at Loma Linda University, in studying the participants of the 1987 Los Angeles Marathon, discovered that 40 percent had experienced the flu or at least one cold during the two months preceding the marathon. Also, the week after the race, 2,300 marathoners caught colds.

Does *excessive* exercise weaken the immune system? If the answer is yes, then why? Research concludes that the most common thread in such cases is intense exercise programs or "distress exercise." Marathon runners subject themselves to the chronic physical fatigue and frequent injuries that often accompany overtraining.

Researchers at Loma Linda University have presented studies indicating that moderate exercise is just as effective as intense training in reducing deaths from all causes and in prolonging life. That is, moderation is the key to healthy exercise and fitness.

We live in a culture that says, "If some is good, more is better." But when you exercise to excess—and excess varies with individuals—you harm your health.

Our research says that healthy, long-lived people observe moderation in everything for most of their lives. When they eat, for instance, they eat small meals. Many of them exercise extensively, but they walk rather than run. They live at a slightly slower pace, yet they feel they accomplish what they need to do. All are flexible people who accept the joys and disappointments in life as expressions of the will of God.

- Dr. Robert Samp at the University of Wisconsin confirmed that almost all long-lived people have a conservative, middle-of-the-road outlook and personality. They take prudent risks but not unnecessary or hazardous ones.

- Dr. Dean Ornish has stated that most degenerative diseases are diseases of excess, caused by eating an overabundance of food or dietary fat; indulging in alcohol, caffeine, or cigarettes; exercising excessively; or developing an extremely stressful response to life events.

- In 1988, Jan presented a longevity paper at the American Public Health Association meetings in Boston. His research showed that men who were 20 percent overweight had a two-year shorter life expectancy than those of normal weight.

Avoid extremes of any kind.

You can even go to extremes in health reform. You can be absolutely correct and rigidly adhere to diet and exercise—and still be miserable. It's been found that those who hate exercise lose much of the benefit. Find a form of exercise you can enjoy.

Don't try to change everything at once. Instead, choose one area and try it. For example, introduce two or three fat-free recipes or low-sugar foods into your diet.

Don't shock your family with too much good at once and risk rejection of all health reform. In everything, keep a positive, optimistic spirit. Be flexible. Laugh at your mistakes. Don't take yourself too seriously.

GETTING PRACTICAL

1. Make gradual changes. If you decide to become a vegetarian, for example, begin by eliminating red meat and continuing to eat poultry and fish for a while.

2. Set small, easily obtainable goals. If you are 40 pounds overweight, don't try to lose all those pounds in four weeks. Ease into a program of reducing food intake and increasing physical exercise.

3. Moderate exercise leaves you feeling healthier and more energetic. If you have to rest for an hour afterward, you are probably overexerting yourself.

4. Moderate means not stressful. If you have to push yourself to do

more, you may want to examine your activity. Ask yourself, Why do I need more?

5. Moderation

- preserves your health

- helps you maintain your energy level

- gives you a sense of having control over your desires

- postpones the occurrence of disease and eliminates some types

- provides the "safety" mechanism when you erroneously adopt any bad health practices

- introduces balance into your life

_____

Moderation positively affects my health,
longevity, and the quality of my life.

FREEBIES FOR YOUR HEALTH

THE SHIP arrived at Antarctica December 24, 1928. Richard Byrd and his crew of forty-one unloaded supplies for Little America—the place they would stay for the next 14 months. When they arrived, the sun shone for 24 hours. As the men worked, they knew time only by checking their watches.

• • •

Then the length of the days began to decrease. In his autobiography, *With Byrd at the Bottom of the World,* Norman Vaughan spoke of the effects of decreasing sunlight. One man became severely morose and depressed: "In April we lost the sun. Now only pale moonlight lightened the twenty-four hours of darkness. The long night of continued and total darkness affects people differently."[1]

For five dark months, they lived in buildings connected by underground tunnels. The morale of the men deteriorated. The sun finally returned on August 20, 1929, and Vaughan writes: "How can I explain the joyousness of the first few days of sunlight? We felt like prisoners who had received commutation of our sentences. A brightness appeared on our faces. We walked faster and moved with an energy we had long forgotten."[2]

Those men had taken the sunlight for granted—until they spent five months without it. Like the men of Byrd's exploratory party, most of us take the sun for granted. Yet it is more than just the light of day.

Modern technology confirms that the sun mediates all life on earth, from the tiniest plants to the human body. Light is the starting place of life. The biblical account of creation says that on the first day God commanded light to appear (see Gen. 1:1–5).

Sunlight provides the environment needed for our existence; it plays a role in photosynthesis, which creates oxygen. Sunlight regulates temperature and humidity at life-supporting levels. Excluding nuclear energy, the sun is the source of 98 percent of the heat energy on the earth.

Spending a little time in the sun every day provides these benefits:

1. *The sun helps to heal certain diseases and prevents infections.* Known as heliotherapy, exposure to sunlight kills germs. We can trace this understanding back more than 2,000 years to Hippocrates, the father of medicine.

2. *The sun provides vitamin D* (really a hormone). Your marvelous body can make this chemical, also found in certain foods, *when sunlight touches your skin.* (The difference between vitamins and hormones is that although they are of similar nature and function, the body can make hormones.)

   Your body needs about 400 units of vitamin D each day. By exposing your face to sunlight for only five minutes daily, you can provide for all the vitamin D you need. What a healthy freebie!

3. *Sunlight gives you healthier skin.* Sunlight enables your skin to resist disease and infections. Proper amounts of sunlight make your skin smooth and pliable, and gives it a healthy glow. Tanned skin is three times more powerful in killing germs than untanned. *However,* too much sunlight can damage the skin and prepare the way for skin cancer. Repeated sunburn dehydrates and wrinkles the skin.

No group of diseases is more extensively treated with light therapy than skin diseases. Acne, psoriasis, pityriasis rosea, and ulceration of the skin, such as that caused by varicose veins, injury, and insect bites, respond well to graded doses of sunlight.

4. *Your nervous system responds favorably to sunlight.* In recent years, research has detected that some people, especially women, suffer from SAD (seasonal affective disorder). Long periods with few hours of light in the winter affect their nerves and emotions.

   Indications are that sunlight increases the endorphins your brain manufactures and gives you a better sense of well-being.

5. *Sunlight strengthens your heart and improves your circulation.* In the cardiovascular system, the benefits of sunlight parallel those of exercise. Like exercise, it lowers the resting pulse rate, tunes up the heart muscle, and increases cardio-output by improving your heart's efficiency. It also tends to normalize your blood pressure, whether it's high or low.

6. *Sunlight builds your immune system.* Your body has several lines of defense that begin with the skin and the mucous membranes. Sunlight enhances your immune system by increasing the oxygen-carrying capacity of the red cells.

7. *Sunlight aids you in losing weight.* By stimulating the thyroid gland to increase hormone productivity, sunshine in turn increases your rate of metabolism and thus helps you burn more calories.

WHAT ABOUT SKIN CANCER?

Sunlight is the major risk factor in skin cancer. The U.S. National Cancer Institute predicts that one of six Americans will develop some form of skin cancer.

Most of the forty thousand new skin cancer cases diagnosed annually in the United States could be prevented if people protected themselves against overexposure to sunlight. Skin pigment, melanin, protects against skin cancer by filtering some of the ultraviolet light that enters your skin. This explains why light-skinned people have more skin cancer than those with darker skins. If you're African-American, you have the most melanin in your skin, and the lowest incidence of skin cancer.

Although most skin cancers are readily curable, malignant melanoma (the most serious and rapid growing) accounts for 75 percent of the 7,400 skin cancer deaths each year. Following breast cancer, skin cancer is the leading cause of cancer in women. Especially vulnerable are those ages twenty-five to twenty-nine.

When you start exposing yourself to the sun, keep this in mind: *Shorter, multiple exposures are better than one lengthy exposure.* The high-risk time for getting sunburned is between 10:00 A.M. and 3:00 P.M. When you must be exposed to the sun for long periods of time, wear protective clothing and put sunscreen lotion on unprotected skin. However, to get the most benefit from the sun, don't overdo the use of sunscreens, oils, or lotions. They keep the oil-secreting glands of your body from working properly. If you do spend large amounts of time in the sun, it's fine to perspire because that cools you and gets rid of body poisons.

Besides skin cancer, research now says that excessive sun exposure causes free radicals to develop in your skin cells. These free radicals are highly destructive molecules that damage tissue, cause premature aging, and can lead to cancer.

BREATHING IT IN

Let's take the next step and talk about how we breathe the air God has provided. You're an aerobic creature, and you need fresh air to sustain life. Every day you take more than 17,000 breaths to keep your body fueled. Human beings can live for weeks without food and days without water, but only minutes without air. For most people, six to eight minutes without oxygen causes irreversible brain damage.

HOW YOU BREATHE IS IMPORTANT

Part of the quality of your life depends on how well you inhale and exhale. If you're typical, you use less than half your lung capacity when breathing. Shallow, improper breathing reduces vitality and causes your metabolic rate to slow down, and can bring on fatigue and exhaustion. It affects memory, creativity, and concentration as well as your judgment and willpower. In extreme cases, it can lead to anemia and depression. If you will habitually inhale and exhale deeper (by using your abdominal muscle), you can help to decrease those symptoms.

YOUR EMOTIONS AND BREATHING

Breathing affects your emotions—something most people don't realize—and, conversely, strong emotional feelings affect your breathing. When you're afraid or extremely nervous, you take rapid, shallow breaths. Grief and anger work the same way. Even happier emotions like joy produce changes in body tension and restrict breathing.

Haven't you had the experience of being startled? hearing a sudden noise in the middle of the night? barely avoiding a serious accident? How do you respond? "My heart is still racing," you say, because it takes several minutes to return to normal.

Tension of any kind alters your normal breathing patterns. Fear increases tension and tension restricts breathing. This shows the intimate relationship between body and mind. If anger continues to stir you and constrict your breathing, it's bound to have some long-term effect on your health!

Strong emotions and shallow breathing go together. Some researchers believe that shallow breathing is learned in infancy. How many times have you watched babies hold their breath? Small children suppress anger by pulling back their shoulders and constricting their chest and throat muscles to prevent screaming. *Suppression of emotion results in muscle tension that limits respiration.*

As you grew toward adulthood and faced more intense stress, repression increased. If you buried your feelings instead of expressing them, that act restricted your breathing, and eventually you developed poor breathing habits.

Such habits can make you prone to develop such negative feelings as anger, depression, and low self-esteem. The corrective measure is for you to learn to breathe freely and naturally.

If you breathe deeply and slowly, it calms you. That's the basis for relaxation techniques.

Help yourself to breathe better by following these tips:

1. Exercise outside, in the mornings when the air is cleanest. Many adults, especially in cold weather, walk inside shopping malls. They would benefit more if they went outside and breathed fresh air.

2. Wear loose-fitting clothing. The tighter the clothes around your waist, the less healthy they are because they tend to constrict breathing.

3. Practice breathing deeply. Breathe from your diaphragm—down at the bottom of your lungs—instead of taking shallow draughts from the top. This will become habitual if you practice.

4. Get to the "second wind." Practice fast exercises, such as running or walking up a hill, so that you get your second wind—the point where heavy exercise no longer makes you feel out of breath.

5. Spend as much time as possible among trees. They are excellent oxygen producers.

BREATHING AND POLLUTION

Despite all we know about pollution, we still take in too much contaminated air. Among the pollutants we breathe in are carbon monoxide, sulfur oxide, sulfates, nitrogen oxide, benzopyrene, ozone, cadmium, and mercury. This contamination comes not only from industrial waste and auto emissions, but also from tobacco smoke. (Of course, polluted air is better than no air.)

Pollution Indoors

We hear increasingly about the need for clean air. As more of us become concerned about pollution, we learn—often to our amazement —just how much dirty air we're inhaling.

Pollutants fill the air outdoors, but indoor pollution is just as serious. Pollutants can be 20 times higher inside homes than outside. Although tobacco smoke remains the most common issue, one report says that the average American household contains a combined total of 63,000 different chemicals, many of which are toxic. Most Americans now spend 90 percent of their time indoors, where they breathe in the poisoned air.

Leaded paint is a problem, especially in houses built before 1950. The U.S. Department of Housing and Urban Development (HUD) suggests that 74 percent of all homes built before 1980 have some amount of lead paint on their walls. Inhaling lead dust can cause significant cellular damage as well as other health problems, especially for infants and small children.

Many building products and household goods use *formaldehyde* as a bonding agent and preservative. Formaldehyde is commonly found in hairsprays, disinfectants, shampoos, lipsticks, toothpaste, eye makeup, nail polish, soap, toilet tissue, perfumes, milk cartons, car bodies, curtains, carpets, insulation, upholstery fabrics, and a variety of pressed-wood products, such as paneling and plywood. It puts the "permanent" in permanent-press clothing and the "strength" in wet-strength paper towels.

Radon, which has been receiving attention during the last few years, is a naturally occurring radioactive gas. It may contaminate as many as 10 percent of American homes. Produced by the breakdown of uranium in rock and soil, radon enters structures through cracks in the foundation. It is odorless and colorless, which makes it difficult to detect. If not detected, it leads to lung damage and cancer. Statistics now cite radon as the second leading cause of lung cancer, led only by cigarette and cigar smoking.

GETTING PRACTICAL

You can help cut the amount of pollution in the air by doing a few practical things:

1. Buy nontoxic household cleaning products.

2. Switch from a wood-burning fireplace to gas.

3. Keep your furnace, humidifier, and air conditioner clean. Service them regularly. Change the filters. Have your air ducts professionally cleaned.

4. Keep your house well ventilated, especially the bedrooms. Crack a window or door each day and let in fresh air. If possible, sleep with your windows open, even if you have to add more covers.

5. Have your house checked for radon. You can do this through your regional office of the EPA.

6. Fill your house with live plants. They absorb carbon dioxide and produce oxygen, which means they help keep your indoor air clean as well as adding color to the decor. Especially, add plants to your bedroom, where a lot of carbon dioxide accumulates each night.

7. Air out your house once a day. Air your bedding in the sun whenever possible to avoid pollution from body odors and gases.

8. Drive less; walk more.

Clean air gives me energy and fewer illnesses.

A WHOLE DAY TO REST?

DURING WORLD War II, the United States and Great Britain sped up the production of war materiels. Many factories shifted to seventy-four-hour workweeks. Before long, owners realized that workers averaged only sixty-six hours of actual work. And factory workers complained about feeling irritable. Morale dropped. Accidents increased. Spoilage soared. Owners soon decreased the workweek.

• • •

In the United States, some factories added more workers, and others introduced three eight-hour shifts instead of increasing the hours of the single shift. What were the results? They had higher production, fewer spoiled items, lower rates of absenteeism, and better morale.

In Great Britain, when they reduced the number of working hours to forty-eight a week (eight-hour days, six days a week), production went up. The British then went so far as to declare a mandatory rest of one day each week and gave their workers two weeks of annual vacation.

People have tried other rhythms. For instance, in 1793, the French adopted a calendar of twelve months of thirty days each. Workers stayed on the job for nine days and rested on the tenth.

After thirteen years, they discontinued that calendar. Workers didn't want to work nine days before getting a day of rest.

These historical illustrations point out an in-built human need to rest from work approximately one day in seven.

Perhaps this sounds to you like a strange, badly outdated custom. You live a fast-paced, stress-filled life. One person actually asked regarding time off, "But what do you do? Doesn't it get boring?" If she wasn't doing something, she felt she was wasting time.

She missed the point of the biblical command. The Sabbath can become a special vacationlike day—a time to put aside work, schedules, and daily commitments. You can rest, relax, refocus, and fellowship with your Creator and with each other.

To ensure it is truly a day of rest, some Christians—obviously a minority—ban newspapers, radio, TV, video games, or any business involvement for that twenty-four-hour period. Others are less strict, but they still agree that by putting aside secular pursuits, the pressures and job tensions decrease or even disappear.

If you take on this health practice, use this one-day-in-seven to contemplate God's special blessings of health and fellowship, recharge your moral batteries, and gain spiritual insight about God's plan for your life. After all, to rest one day in seven is one of God's Ten Commandments. (See Exod. 20:8–11.)

> If you choose to live a healthier lifestyle, you can't afford to overlook the important principle of resting one day in seven. On this day, stop your busyness for twenty-four hours.

As much as you think you don't have enough time, you can learn to set aside one day out of seven. This habitual rest provides a basis for a relatively stress-free environment. Seek solitude in the out-of-doors and avoid stress-producing noise. Avoid jammed freeways, shopping malls, packed stadiums, competitive sports to maintain healthier blood pressure levels.

When you say, "I don't have time for a day of rest every week," it's as if you are saying, "I am too busy to obey God and too busy to take care of myself."

The one-in-seven day is a time to cease from work, but it's more. It's also time to step back from accomplishment, from worry and tension, from trying to control your own life. This is an important concept. You and I live in a world where we constantly strive to be in the driver's seat. We want everything done our way. We want to make our world conform to our desires.

For too many people, even though they're not physically on the job, the Sabbath is still a busy day—it's just a different kind of busyness. Do you have such a hectic schedule of activities for the Sabbath that you never have the chance to rest? As you rush from one activity to another, do you find you seldom enjoy any of them because of the time factor?

We live in a paradoxical time. We have increased goods, timesaving gadgets, more communication tools, and faster means of transportation. Yet most of us also probably have much higher rates of physical exhaustion, emotional frustration, social neglect, and inner restlessness.

Those who follow this principle of resting consistently show by their lifestyles that they have something important that others lack: a weekly, twenty-four-hour downtime. Aside from the spiritual value they gain, they give themselves a rest from the overstimulation of their bodies' adrenal system, which most of them understand as the root of many modern stress problems.

If Sabbath observance is one of the major reasons some people live a decade longer and healthier, isn't that reason enough to give it a good try?

Stop.

Quit working for one full day.

Rest.

Give yourself a true Sabbath.

The root of the word *Sabbath* means "to stop, rest, cease." This refers to God's acts of creation. After bringing the world into being,

God stopped, not from tiredness, but because the work was finished. This is the reasoning behind the command to observe the Sabbath. Adherents of this biblical principle believe that God intended them to "finish" their work for the week.

Those who follow the Live-Longer Lifestyle emphasize that observing the Sabbath *isn't a legalistic duty*—although some may treat it as such. Rather, it's living in accordance with our natural rhythm, which gives us freedom and relief from stress.

Perhaps a better way to look at this matter is to concentrate on the *purpose* behind the command. Why did God give this command to the people? Was it merely to make them "different" or was it done for their good?

Those who follow the command to rest one day a week believe it wasn't merely an arbitrary order. God sanctified (set apart) that day for the good of humanity. History has shown this rhythm fits human life. If the command to rest one day out of seven is for the good of the human race, then ponder carefully the implications of saying no to this strong Old Testament command.

The Live-Longer Lifestyle research indicates that those who literally set aside time for rest

- experience less hypertension
- feel less stress
- have fewer divorces
- have fewer suicides

Here are five reasons to incorporate a day of rest into your life.

1. *Your body needs rest.* You can't keep on giving without pausing to restore. To fully observe this practice means to refrain from ordinary work—including even thoughts of ordinary work. You can, however, engage in joyful activities, the things that do you good and make you feel you have gained inwardly from

the experience. This could mean taking your family hiking in the mountains, spending an uninterrupted period reading, taking a long solitary walk in the woods. The idea is that it is a time to cease from normal activities.

2. *What you spend your time on reveals your true priorities.* The Sabbath provides you with a weekly opportunity to serve God. Although you may serve God every day, Sabbath means you desist from gainful employment and secular pursuits in order to honor God. To rest deliberately is to serve God.

   Those of us who see this as guidance for today believe that God asks us to withdraw from daily pressures to meet with God in the quietness of our souls. This shows our love, loyalty, and devotion to God. We willingly tune out hundreds of voices that demand attention so we can be in tune with God.

   One man likes to say, "If you observe the Sabbath, you offer God the devotion of your total being."

3. *The Sabbath provides you with opportunities to consider others.* Why not make this day of rest a time when you shift the focus away from yourself?

   Of the Ten Commandments, the fourth is the only one that goes into detail about other people: sons and daughters, servants and sojourners, even animals. God created this as a day for all—not just for a chosen few.

   Many think about the needy on the Sabbath or the "stranger within your gates" (Exod. 23:12; Deut. 5:14). They see this as an opportunity to share food and friendship with widows, orphans, the elderly, the estranged and discouraged people in the church and community.

4. *A weekly day for rest means service to yourself.* Many who follow this principle speak of being enriched when they rest and worship God. They receive strength and vitality by not working. This

becomes a day of reflection, a time to review the week and learn from their restlessness. For them the Sabbath involves more than attending a place of worship—it provides both space and time to meditate, to let their minds dwell on spiritual realities.

In our modern world most of us tend to base our self-worth on our level of productivity. During this day of rest, you can remind yourself that you are loved just because you were created by God. Working harder or longer doesn't make you more—or less—loved. By the simple act of refraining from work at least fifty-two days each year, you remind yourselves that God doesn't demand us to be productive every minute and every day.

This day provides you with time to be close to the special people in your life. Call a halt to the rushed activities of the week and say, "Today is a day for my family." Such an attitude strengthens families and relationships.

One person remarked, "Observing the Sabbath has liberated me. I don't have to be in control of everything around me. It is my time to let go and simply enjoy life."

5. *A day of rest reminds you that you are part of this world and responsible for it.* "The land is mine and you are . . . my tenants" (Lev. 25:23 NIV). As you contemplate the meaning of this day, you can learn to acknowledge God's ownership of this world. You learn not to misuse or exploit nature because it is God's handiwork. (See Ps. 19:1.) Stand back and celebrate the grandeur and mystery of creation and life.

In the New Testament, Jesus said that the Sabbath was made for humanity, not for humanity to slavishly follow a law (see Mark 2:27). He also said that it was a day to do good (Matt. 12:12), to save (Mark 3:4), to free people from physical and spiritual bondage (Luke 13:12–16), and to show mercy (Matt. 12:7).

Above all, the Sabbath rest is not just a day off from work.
To think in such a way focuses on utilitarianism. It's not about wasting time or *not* working. It's a different kind of time. Observing this weekly break makes all activities—participation in informal fellowship and recreation as well as participation in formal worship—offerings to God.

If you observe a weekly day of rest, you can

- become more aware of God's creative power and love for the human race
- realize your responsibility to protect God's creation from pollution
- depend more fully on divine power to offer guidance
- cultivate spiritual growth
- strengthen family relationships and friendships
- improve habits of loving and helping others
- appreciate a sensible, balanced lifestyle
- learn to cope with anxiety, depression, and fear, and to control anger
- develop a stronger sense of self-esteem and self-confidence

GETTING PRACTICAL

Once you acknowledge these benefits, it still requires planning to make setting aside one day a weekly experience. Try these tips.

1. Establish a deliberate beginning and ending to your twenty-four hours.

2. Make a conscious decision to observe this day. It won't "just happen"—it's something you must decide on *and plan for*. It takes preparation to get essential things done before the Sabbath hours (such as heavy cooking, house cleaning, or yard work) so you can relax without being constantly reminded of things you need to do.

3. Make the day significantly different from the other six days in your week. If you watch TV, read newspapers, listen to radio, or sit at your computer on a daily basis, change your routine. Substitute healthful activities. Making the day significantly different will ensure not only bodily rest, but mental rest as well.

4. Make it clear to your friends and family members that you have made this commitment. Many people report how cooperative loved ones become once they recognize the principles by which they live. Friends may not agree, but they'll probably respect you for living your values. As they see the beneficial results in your life, they may even want to join you.

5. Accept that you'll have conflicts. If you hold to the observance of a rest day, you will need to guard it and, except in times of humanitarian need, refuse to participate in the normal activities of modern life.

6. Remind yourself that you commit yourself to observing the Sabbath because it is a significant factor in healthier, stress-free living.

---

*Because I choose to live longer and healthier,
I observe a full day of rest every week.*

MAKING THE RIGHT MOVES

CHAPTER 20

ARE YOU convinced you want to change your lifestyle?

• • •

Are you committed to living longer and healthier?

If you answer yes, this is the most important chapter for you. You are at the point of making a decision that will affect the rest of your life.

One way to show you that following the Live-Longer Lifestyle can enable you to live healthier and longer is to give you the results of a study on health practices.

Jan and his colleagues gleaned a lot of information from the work of Dr. Lester Breslow and his team, who surveyed nearly seven thousand residents of Alameda County in northern California. They asked the residents a variety of questions, such as whether they smoked, exercised, were overweight, ate breakfast, slept seven or eight hours a night, and snacked between meals. The survey also asked the subjects about their consumption of alcohol.

After following the group for nine years, the team learned that 38 percent of the men ages sixty to sixty-nine who adopted no more than two of the health practices had died. By comparison, of those who had adopted four or five practices, only 24 percent had died.

For women, 38 percent who adopted no more than two had died, while only 9 percent of those who adopted four or five had died. This

study shows that anyone—even after age sixty—who adopts good
health practices can decrease the risk of dying prematurely from such
major diseases as heart disease, cancer, and stroke.

MAKING THE CHANGES

Altering your health habits, particularly the way you eat, means
doing away with long-established habits. Making the adjustments won't
be easy, but you can make them—regardless of your age. Those of us
who work with people who want to make changes know you have to
be persistent (and often creative).

That will be the first, difficult step for you—sticking with your
commitment to improve your health. Remind yourself that it usually
takes concentrated effort for at least three weeks before the new habits
become entrenched. If you persist, by then you should also see wonderful progress toward your ultimate goals.

Follow these steps to change your lifestyle:

1. *Prepare.* Educate yourself, as you are doing through reading this
   book. Continue to read and learn how you can take control of
   your health for quality living. Remember, you are *not* implement-
   ing a diet—a program of restriction—but changing your lifestyle.
   Let your plan include occasional permission to eat something that
   you typically wouldn't touch with your new way of eating.

   Allowing such breaks will help you to feel less deprived,
   which, in the long run, can help you adapt to your new lifestyle.

   Anticipate problems, such as giving in to snacking opportunities, overeating at a dinner party, handling stressful situations
   poorly, or trying to excuse yourself from walking when it's rain-
   ing. Visualize resourceful and appropriate solutions—then,
   when these situations do occur, you will have a plan in place.
   Visualizing yourself as one who is successfully adopting changes
   can be an effective tool in your growth.

2. *Say these words to yourself each day:*

> Because I want to live longer and healthier, I will stick with my lifestyle changes at least twenty-one days.

3. *Choose one health practice at a time* whether it's reducing your weight, drinking eight glasses of water daily, exercising, or giving up snacking or smoking. Why not select the least difficult first? A series of small victories can prepare you for the major changes.

4. *Set small, weekly goals you can achieve.* Make a chart so you can monitor your progress. For example, if you choose to drink more water, set goals for the number of glasses you plan to drink each day the first week and keep track of how well you meet your goals.

   Every success—no matter how small—enables you to move toward a healthier and longer life.

5. *Be moderate.* You don't have to achieve everything at once. If you wish to adopt the vegetarian lifestyle, start with one vegetarian meal a week. Don't force the change on your family. Choose recipes that taste so good that family members want more. *Use this approach in every change you decide to make.*

6. *List your ultimate goals as accomplished.* They could read like this:

   • I enjoy better health and avoid many illnesses because I have adopted the major health practices in this book.

   • I manage my weight better.

   • I respond to stressful events in healthy ways.

   • I get the amount of sleep I need.

   • I have improved my diet.

- I apply the principles of moderation in everything I do.

Once you decide on and list your ultimate goals, you'll need to review them regularly.

Keep your goals in your mind when you are tempted to give in. Visualize yourself as successful in attaining each one. Many athletes use visualization techniques to successfully reach their goals—and you can too. Think of how it will feel when you achieve a goal. Think of the better quality of your life. Think about the money you will save by adopting these goals and what you want to do with it.

Yes, you are in charge, and yes, it is worth "going for the gold"!

7. *Reward yourself for your achievements.* Enjoy your successes, no matter how small they may seem. Even if it's as simple as drinking two glasses of water a day when you previously drank none. Say to yourself, "This is progress."

Do something really kind for yourself—something you enjoy, such as going to see a play or taking a bubble bath. Avoid food rewards—that promotes bad habits and negative thought patterns.

8. *Forgive yourself when you fail.* Get back on your program as soon as possible (certainly within twenty-four hours). Don't let derailments be permanent. Remind yourself that nobody is perfect and you are making progress. Remember, you are interested in progress, not mistakes, so don't be too hard on yourself.

9. *Monitor your progress daily and review your charts on a weekly basis.* Learn where you need to improve and commend yourself for what you have accomplished.

> Because I want to live healthier and longer, I will persist.

10. *Motivate yourself.* Post notes around the house, the office, and inside

your car to remind yourself of your goals and progress. Avoid areas where you will likely succumb. For example, if snacking is a problem, stay out of the kitchen between 3:00 and 5:00 P.M.

11. *Get support.* Don't try to do it all alone. Before you begin to change, ask friends and family members to help.

12. *Claim your ultimate Resource.* If you are a Christian, you have an additional resource—an important one—God's willingness to help you achieve success. "I can do everything through [Jesus Christ] who gives me strength," wrote the apostle Paul (Phil. 4:13 NIV).

You may want to choose a number of "power" verses from the Bible and keep them accessible to read or repeat when you're facing a temptation. Such verses can be an important tool on your road to a successful lifestyle change.

When you're tempted to quit your exercise program, for example, remember the promise, "No testing has overtaken you that is not common to everyone. God is faithful, and he will not let you be tested beyond your strength . . ." (1 Cor. 10:13 NRSV).

When you push your cart past the candy bars at the supermarket, repeat, "So whether you eat or drink or whatever you do, do it all for the glory of God" (1 Cor. 10:31 NIV).

FINAL THOUGHTS

By now, you have realized that good health is the result of making choices that involve your mind and spirit. You have learned that it's up to you to change—probably to a larger degree than you first realized.

Changes are rarely easy. It takes effort and commitment to get yourself out of a rut and try something new. As you maintain moderate progress, however, you will give yourself reason to believe you can implement even more changes.

Eventually, you'll experience a higher level of health. Your friends can benefit as well if you sensitively share what you have learned. Because you'll feel better, you will treat others better. You may be inspired with new ideas. You may even enjoy the satisfaction that comes from helping others. Your friends will see that you have become a new person.

"Dear friend, I am praying that all is well with you and that your body is as healthy as I know your soul is" (3 John 2 NLT).

I have chosen to live longer and healthier.
I will make gradual changes to my lifestyle.

Lifestyle Centers that promote the Live-Longer Lifestyle with health information seminars and residential programs are located throughout the world. For a current list of these facilities or for other information and resourses that promote the Live-Longer Lifestyle:

- call 1-800-PSALM23 (772-5623)

- visit us on the Web at www.tccm.org

FASTING: THE NEGLECTED HEALTH FACTOR

The health practice least frequently used is fasting. By the term *fast*, we mean abstaining from any food or liquid other than water. (While some take pure juices when fasting to provide vitamins and other nutrients, *fasting properly means ingesting nothing but water.*)

Fasting involves drinking large quantities of water. We suggest that those who undertake a fast think of water intake as a flushing process. The more you take in during the noneating period, the more impurities you flush from your system.

How appealing is this practice to most people? Going without food for a single day, let alone for an extended period, is more than most people even want to think about. This reaction makes it easy to understand why fasting hasn't become a popular health option.

Our culture also works against this practice. We're bombarded daily with TV ads on snacks, diets, and food choices. We can hardly pick up a magazine or a newspaper without seeing pictures of something to eat.

In this time and in this culture, it may seem strange that people actually do choose to fast. Even more surprising is that those who fast regularly do it enthusiastically. If asked, they're usually eager to testify to the derived benefits. Yet most of us either don't try to fast or have tried it and couldn't handle the food deprivation and loss of energy, resultant weakness, or minor physical symptoms, such as headache or nausea.

"Why would I want to fast?" is the question we hear most often when this topic arises. "Who wants to feel tired and miserable all the time?"

Fasting needs to be a deliberate choice. We don't believe in making any demands about such a practice. Not everyone seems suited to do this.

"I went without food once for sixteen hours," reported one man, "and I felt miserable the whole time."

"I tried to fast once," said another person. "I started the day fine, but by one o'clock, I couldn't handle the hunger pains any longer. I gave in."

They then felt guilty for having failed and condemned themselves for lack of willpower or commitment. That's not the purpose of this appendix. Our purpose is to point out that healthy, vibrant people sometimes fast, some as frequently as one day a week.

So why should anyone fast? Devotees of the fast offer three reasons:

1. *They fast for improved health.* This means, primarily, enhanced health. Fasting isn't starvation. Going without food for periods of time actually brings about health benefits. Some begin fasting as soon as they have the first symptoms of a cold or fever. Not eating allows the digestive organs to rest and speeds up the elimination of toxins from the body. Putting all its energy into recuperation allows the body to heal itself.

   We know from observing the animal world that fasting is a natural, normal process. Haven't most of us observed an animal that wouldn't take food when wounded or sick? Many humans instinctively lose their appetites and want nothing to eat when they're unwell. That's therapeutic fasting.

   Fasting is also an ancient form of hygiene, still practiced in many cultures. Fasting temporarily stops the accumulation of matter to be digested and allows the body to rest from the work of digestion and catch up with the process of cleansing.

   Fasting is a good way to withdraw from the use of alcohol, nicotine, caffeine, or even prescription drugs. When we become accustomed to certain ingested stimulants and then remove them, our bodies argue with us about the deprivation, and we feel uncomfortable and miserable. The most common complaints associated with fasting are headaches, weakness, and nausea; but the practice provides ideal conditions for the body to regenerate, repair, and rejuvenate itself.

2. *They fast to lose weight.* Some refer to the twenty-four-hour fast as a secret weapon. For people who either have a lot of weight to lose or who want to get rid of pounds in a hurry, it has proved effective. *However, fasting one meal a day (such as not eating supper) is the most effective "fast" for weight loss.* (A number of people, unable to lose weight permanently by traditional methods, have found that fasting from the completion of their noon meal until breakfast is an excellent weight-reduction program.)

On short fasts—up to three days—people can lose weight. But they do not lose much on a prolonged fast. One fasting guru insists that prolonged fasts actually force us to gain. After two or three days, the wise body defends itself by slowing down the metabolism. The longer you fast, the more energy-conserving your body becomes. This means that because your system slows down, prolonged fasting for weight loss is counterproductive.

3. *They fast for spiritual reasons.* Jesus *assumed* that people fasted. He said, "When you fast, do not look somber as the hypocrites do. . . . But when you fast, put oil on your head and wash your face" (Matt. 6:16–17 NIV).

Since ancient times, people have seen fasting as a form of self-humbling, when combined with prayer, or as a physical retreat from others. A number of verses in the Bible refer to fasting, for example, 2 Samuel 12:16–23; Ezra 8:21; Psalm 69:10–11; Isaiah 58:5–7; Jonah 3:7.

Here are a few of the spiritual reasons to fast:

- to present a petition before God
- to demonstrate the seriousness of the request
- to more fully praise, worship, and honor God
- to receive spiritual insight or direction
- to develop self-discipline

If you decide to fast:

1. Examine your motivation. Why do you want to fast? Be clear about what you want to achieve.

2. Think of it as a positive action—something you want to do for yourself. (Remember that you already fast each night while you sleep. Fasting extends the noneating period of time into the waking hours.)

3. Prepare by cutting out snacks. Take nothing but water between meals. Once you have learned to do this comfortably, it means you have already gone without food for four to six hours between breakfast and lunch and again from lunch until dinner. You have taken your first steps toward fasting!

4. Consider eating only two meals a day by cutting out the evening meal. The principle, as mentioned elsewhere, is to eat breakfast like a king (making it the biggest meal of the day), lunch like a queen, and the evening meal like a pauper. If you follow this plan, your next step would be to cut out the evening meal altogether.

   Those who follow the two-meals-a-day plan do it because they believe it is better for the digestive system and the body processes. You give your stomach longer rest periods.

This practice will demand self-discipline. You probably grew up eating three meals a day at prescribed times of day. You may not find it easy to change such long-standing habits.

BREAKING THE FAST

If you go on a one-day fast, you may not have any difficulty in returning to normal (i.e., healthy) eating. However, especially if you have not fasted before, you may want to begin with pure fruit juices to break the fast. Not everyone agrees with this. Some suggest going immediately to whole foods to activate the salivary glands and re-establish bowel function more rapidly. Let your own sense of hunger guide you.

Fasting is perhaps the ultimate demonstration of being in charge of your health because it requires you to deny the hunger urge that drives many people to overindulge.

Unless there are other health problems, such as diabetes or hypoglycemia, anyone can fast safely for one day. Some people set aside one day each week for total abstinence from anything but water.

Fasting for a day will not only help you burn off damaged fat cells and cleanse your body of a number of toxins, but it can also help you experience incredible physical and spiritual health benefits. If you have the courage, you might like to try it.

Whether I fast or not, I take charge of my health.

THE BIBLE: RECORDED LONG AGO

"It says in the Bible," is one way many Christians begin in affirming their beliefs. And it's more than just "somewhere in the Bible"; those believers can often quote the book, chapter, and verse. They can do this because biblical principles are the basis of their religious faith, but we can also go to the Bible's pages to gain understanding of health. The health message of the Live-Longer Lifestyle comes from texts that state that our bodies belong to God our Creator. Here are three of them:

- "So whether you eat or drink or whatever you do, do it all for the glory of God" (1 Cor. 10:31 NIV).

- "Therefore, I urge you, brothers, in view of God's mercy, to offer your bodies as living sacrifices . . ." (Rom. 12:1 NIV).

- "Do you not know that your body is a temple of the Holy Spirit, who is in you, whom you have received from God? You are not your own; you were bought at a price. Therefore honor God with your body" (1 Cor. 6:19–20 NIV; see also 3:16).

The Bible teaches us that we have a moral responsibility to live according to the Creator's directives. As more people embrace the Live-Longer Lifestyle, they also begin to shun any practice that weakens the vigor and stamina of their minds or bodies.

When people search for more meaningful, healthier, and longer lives, we hope they also acknowledge more than the physical element of health and sickness. We've long understood that our minds play a significant role in our health and well-being. Now some researchers are extending that concept as they realize the importance of spiritual values in human lives.

We believe the spiritual realm is basic in our orientation to life and health. For example, the admonition and promise for health can be seen in Proverbs 3:1–2 and 8: "My son, do not forget my teaching, but keep my commands in your heart, for they will prolong your life many years and bring you prosperity. . . . This will bring health to your body and nourishment to your bones" (NIV).

With that background, we want to go to the Bible itself as the source for the health practices we try to follow.

Plant-based diet. Many Christians believe that vegetarianism was God's "original diet." Scientific evidence indicates that the original diet provided all the essential nutritive properties necessary to make good blood and fortify the immune system with killer T-cells to fight cancer and other disease invaders.

Genesis 1:29 presents this diet: "I have provided all kinds of fruit and grain for you to eat" (CEV). Genesis 7:2 and 9:3–4 distinguish between clean and unclean animals. Leviticus 3:17 says God's people shouldn't eat fat or blood. Numbers 11:7–8 says that God provided manna for food during the Jews' wilderness wanderings. (Read Exod. 16:2–36.) Exodus 15:26 gives instructions to keep healthy. (See also Deut. 7:12; Jer. 30:17.)

Leviticus 11:1–40 and Ezekiel 4:9 are Old Testament dietary laws, which we believe are valid for healthy living today. Especially see the story of Daniel (Dan. 1:8–21), who refused to eat meat and rich foods and remained healthy by eating vegetables.

Alcohol. Despite some recent health claims about the benefit of moderate alcohol use, many verses warn against intoxicating beverages: Proverbs 20:1; 23:31–32; Isaiah 5:22; 1 Samuel 25:36–38;

Esther 1; Daniel 5. Genesis 19:30–38 relates the story of Lot getting drunk and committing incest.

Rest and relaxation. "Come aside by yourselves to a deserted place and rest a while" (Mark 6:31 NKJV) is a text Jan sometimes uses when he becomes stressed out or aware that he needs a change of pace. (See Ps. 46:10.)

Jesus also said, "One does not live by bread alone, but by every word that comes from the mouth of God" (Matt. 4:4 NRSV).

One of the favorite texts concerning health is, "A cheerful heart is good medicine, but a crushed spirit dries up the bones" (Prov. 17:22 NIV). See also Psalm 16:11; 37:5, 7; Matthew 6:25, 27, 32–33; 10:31; Luke 12:22–30; 2 Corinthians 4:16–17; Jeremiah 29:11.

Moderation. "So whether you eat or drink or whatever you do, do it all for the glory of God" (1 Cor. 10:31 NIV). See also Isaiah 5:11.

Relationships. Proper relationships with others and with God are of primary importance. Good spiritual health helps us and others to practice the Golden Rule: "In everything do to others as you would have them do to you; for this is the law and the prophets" (Matt. 7:12 NRSV; cf. Rom. 12:9–19).

Prayer. "The LORD is near to all who call on him, to all who call on him in truth. He fulfills the desires of those who fear him; he hears their cry and saves them" (Ps. 145:18–19 NIV). See also Matthew 7:7; 21:22; James 5:14–15.

NOTES

2. GET AN ATTITUDE!

1. As quoted by Dale Carnegie, *How to Stop Worrying and Start Living* (New York: Simon & Schuster, 1948), 253–54.

2 Lee S. Berk et al., "Neuroendocrine and Stress Hormone Changes During Mirthful Laughter," *The American Journal of the Medical Sciences* 298, no. 6. (Dec. 1989): 390.

3. Marianne K. Hering, "Believe Well, Live Well," *Focus on the Family* (Sept. 1994): 2–4.

4. Norman Vincent Peale, *How to Make Positive Imaging Work for You* (Rawling, New York: Foundations of Christian Living Publications, 1982).

9. A STOP IN TIME

1. C. Everett Koop, *Surgeon General's 1990 Report* (Washington, D.C.: U.S. Government Printing Office, 1990), xi.

16. MOBILIZING DEFENSES

1. Dean Ornish, *Love and Survival* (New York: HarperCollins, 1998), 131.

18. FREEBIES FOR YOUR HEALTH

1. Norman D. Vaughn with Cecil B. Murphey, *With Byrd at the Bottom of the World* (Harrisburg, Penn.: Stackpole Books, 1990), 57.

2 Ibid., 93.

ABOUT THE AUTHORS

Jan W. Kuzma is a long-time specialist in issues of lifestyle and longevity. The founding chairman of the Department of Biostatistics and former Director of Research for the Loma Linda University School of Public Health, he spent eight years overseeing the study that forms the basis of this book. He now serves as president of a private statistical consulting firm, writes material for a daily radio program, *Got a Minute for Your Health?* and pens a column for the health magazine *Vibrant Life*. He is coauthor of a daily inspirational book, *Energized*.

Cecil Murphy is an award-winning and widely published writer—the author or coauthor of more than seventy books in such wide-ranging fields as health and fitness, motivation, travel, celebrity biography, and inspiration.